A Year of Ebola:

Durable lessons; and, essays on our ancient relationship with infectious diseases

Written by: David M. Brett-Major

Published by,

Navigating Health Risks, LLC

Omaha, Nebraska

www.navigatinghealthrisks.com

ISBN: 978-0-9983651-6-9 (0-9983651-6-5)

Table of Contents

A Year of Ebola: Forward to the 2024 edition 5
Introduction 18
Being at WHO 26
Chapter 1—On assignment to WHO 28
Chapter 2—A very fast primer on WHO, and Ebola 31
WHO 31
Ebola virus 34
Guinea 38
Chapter 3—Conakry and learning about clinical/public health divides 40
Chapter 4—Working inside the Donka Hospital Ebola treatment unit 69
Sierra Leone 82
Chapter 5—Home in Geneva 84
Chapter 6—Kenema 92
Chapter 7—More patients and less staff 111
Photos 153
Nigeria 167
Chapter 8—A brief respite 169
Chapter 9—Lagos 176
Ending in Geneva 208
Chapter 10—Anti-climax 210
Navy, health security, and insider politics 221
Chapter 11—Epilogue 223
Essays on our ancient relationship with infectious diseases 244
Learned fear, and a short history of the plagues 244

What does a healthy relationship look like?..........247
Communication and honesty..........247
Respect, trust, and equality..........253
Mutual choices, economic partnering, and joint parenting..........256
Who are lepers?..........258
Measles is bad. Vaccines are good...........264
Follow the money (or, health is not all about health)..........268
What is next after COVID-19?..........271
About the Author..........275
Letter to the Adadevoh Health Trust..........276

A Year of Ebola: Forward to the 2024 edition

The initial print edition of *A Year of* Ebola was published in 2016. Why a new edition now? Firstly, I have been nagged by colleagues to join the modern age that favors audio books. Secondly, all of us now have a recent, shared health disaster experience, the novel coronavirus 2019 (COVID-19) pandemic.

Severe Acute Respiratory Syndrome coronavirus-2 (SARS-CoV-2) emerged in late 2019. As of August, 2023, the World Health Organization attributed almost 7 million deaths to its spread—this likely has grossly underestimated burden and consequence. Many of these deaths were preventable with usual respiratory risk management measures such as physical and social distancing; distributed, high-fidelity testing coupled with proactive surveillance; mask use; personal and environmental hygiene; and, vaccination and targeted therapies. Among the many survivors of more severe disease, debility is common. Some persons who experienced less severe COVID-19 have long term consequences, as well. Much of this was predictable. Yet, often in the COVID-19 pandemic we did not apply old, well-understood lessons to ensure better outcomes; rather, we made choices in personal and collective behavior that increased household and community cost from a rapidly emerged, pervasive threat to life and wellness, a threat that was not the least bit subtle in its onset or consequences.

For a time after I wrote *A Year of Ebola*, I thought that I had made unique observations on the disconnects between what we know about managing emerging diseases risks and how we act in health-related emergencies and disasters. Of course, little knowledge is new, or as I more often say, all knowledge is old. Later, I read two interesting biographies which I commend to you, *The Medical Detective* by Sandra Hempel and *Benjamin Rush* by Stephen Fried. Written about 19th century Dr. John Snow and 18th century Dr. Benjamin Rush, I experienced morbid humor and exasperation reading the similarities of challenges in mobilizing sensible, concerted community action and the experiences of health emergency and disaster risk managers today—forget for a moment Rush's penchant for overuse of leeches. These two physicians were astonishingly human and accomplished individuals with fascinating stories; the books are good reads.

These risk management disconnects happen frequently. Outbreaks are not centennial events. They happen in small and large ways often, allowing difficult habits to develop and be reinforced. The COVID-19 pandemic and other emergencies highlight the importance of bridging our hard-earned experiences and lessons for effective health emergency and disaster risk management to each new threat. And, they serve to reinforce some critical aspects that readers will revisit when reading this book.

1. Keeping patients and communities at the center of decision making is hard for everyone, including health workers.
2. Emergencies like politics are local.
3. Compassion is impactful.

1—Keeping patients and communities at the center. To do this, work must occur across the clinical and public health interface, and the larger ways that communities thrive must be taken into account. In October 2017, I was in Uganda with colleagues. We were traveling to support a research project intended to be in place in advance of a health emergency, so that medical countermeasures can be tested quickly and then applied usefully in patient care. Professor James Lawler conceived of the idea for the project and launched it with a range of partners. It was run by excellent Ugandan scientists at the Infectious Diseases Institute and the Walter Reed Project, both under the auspices of Makerere University in Kampala. Because of this work, we were known entities to the Ugandan public health enterprise and were asked to visit Kapchorwa and Kween near Mount Elgon as they learned of a Marburg outbreak in those locations. Uganda has a fair amount of experience with filovirus outbreaks from Ebola and Marburg viruses, with small ones occurring as often as every few years.

When we arrived in Kapchorwa, the larger of the two locales, several days after the initial cases, the response team was well organized with the usual leadership elements, such as surveillance and case management including coordination with the Uganda Virus Research Institute, environmental hygiene and logistics, risk communication and social mobilization, and administration and finance. The hospital, however, had not yet been organized to safely manage cases. As we provided some training, our colleagues Saima Zaman and Michael Kozlowski made runs to local markets to get supplies for implementing unidirectional flow in their infection prevention and control (IPC) practice, so that healthcare providers tending the needs of suspected and confirmed patients with Marburg disease would move from lower risk to higher risk areas in one direction, mitigating transmission in the hospital to other patients and healthcare workers, until reaching an exit lane in which they would decontaminate and remove their personal protective equipment under observation. In contrast, when we arrived at smaller Kween, a defunct health clinic already had been transformed into a site for accepting patients into isolation. They were conducting IPC training, establishing clinic procedures, and digging pits to burn medical waste, if required. However, preparations for seeking cases in the community and coordinating broader action were more limited. In each case, there was good initial work by the Ugandans, though that work was either public health action or clinical action in either place, not yet both.

In September, 2018, and August, 2019, as the Democratic Republic of Congo (DRC) had enlarging Ebola virus disease emergencies, my brief experiences in communities and refugee camps just inside the Ugandan side of the border was similar. In 2018, Dr. Elizabeth

Schnaubelt and I visited a large refugee settlement that had its own robustly staffed surveillance work cell with good data management. While they were cognizant that careful IPC workflows were necessary to conduct safe and effective care, they had not established any such procedures nor the necessary infrastructure to do so. The camp organizers were very knowledgeable about the communities. They worked hard to provide basic health services, and they understood the ways that people who live in the settlement interact with communities back across the DRC border. They were aware, for instance, of mini-bus charters between the settlement and market areas near the outbreak in DRC. However, this had not led to a strategy for prioritizing how to look for imported Ebola disease cases, nor resulted in functional plans for managing instances when people were sick and may have been exposed to the disease. We provided *ad hoc* training and consultation to them; assessed a suspect case with fever and bleeding; and, set up a rudimentary process over the course of the clinical evaluation. This was not ideal and difficult for them to sustain. Fortunately, there were good sepsis (severe infection) and IPC training programs based out of the Infectious Diseases Institute in Kampala to which we referred them afterwards. I have similar stories in the post-West Africa Ebola virus disease epidemic period in Liberia and Nigeria.

In the fall of 2022 during Uganda's Ebola disease Sudan emergency, my colleague Dr. Jana Broadhurst (experienced with Ebola virus disease risk management in Sierra Leone), James, and I saw similar challenges but also benefits of some applied lessons. Their command and control processes were clearly defined; and, they simultaneously were addressing the on-going COVID-19 pandemic. However, there were striking unmet patient needs at the healthcare points where patients most commonly presented initially for care.

The divide between public health and clinical care remains a persistent theme across hundreds of years. Each of Snow's, Rush's, ours, and many others' experiences demonstrate how leadership that is intent in remaining focused on patient and community interests across these and other divides; diverse, resilient, and prepared people; and, resources such as money and supply all must be present and affirmatively applied in order to achieve the best results.

2—Emergencies like politics are local. Part of the work that we all must do is to promote vigilance and the business case that early action and transparency make things better. For instance, another complicating feature of the 2017 Uganda Marburg disease outbreak was that the country was hosting the ministerial meeting of the Global Health Security Agenda. The active emergency response served to highlight Ugandan capabilities in an international spotlight; but, there was little motivation to find cases and hint at gaps. In Kapchorwa, I interviewed an ill healthcare provider who had cared for one of the first cases in the outbreak. I think that the individual probably had Marburg disease. However, I had limited success motivating the response team to consider the person a suspect case. Shortly before that emergency, Uganda had undergone a change in how a declaration of a public health emergency occurred. It required Presidential action, rather than health or disaster authorities. In some instances, such a change bringing public health action up from the Ministry of Health to the Head of State might encourage whole-of-government mindfulness in health security. And, it may have done this generally for the country. In this case, however, it exacerbated the challenges in encouraging aggressive action. Fortunately, thanks to the Uganda core response team, local efforts, some minor international partner support, and a large amount of luck, the Marburg disease outbreak stayed small.

Nonetheless, the GAF problem (G-A-F, you will have to sort what that acronym means) has continued to echo. Interest in Ebola virus disease case finding was episodic across the border from the DRC Ebola emergency in 2018-20—sometimes aggressive when managed by experienced technical groups on site, other times avoidant with reticence to scale broad-based testing. Who wants to be associated with a highly consequential emerging infectious disease event receiving international attention that may point to disparities and unrest? These kinds of difficulties happen everywhere in the world. We experienced a similar challenge in the United States with SARS-CoV-2, more from populist choices than force of law or any real sense of embarrassment.

All of this brings us to the current SARS-CoV-2 pandemic and the single aspect that surprised me as it evolved.

3—Compassion is impactful. Each community has its value and strengths. At the beginning of the COVID-19 pandemic, I thought that fundamental advantages in wealth and resources would make a difference in how the United States would experience the emergency. I was not at all surprised by what SARS-CoV-2 does biologically or from a focused epidemiologic perspective. However, I was very surprised by our own apathy and the challenges in demonstrating consideration of others.

In Kenema, Sierra Leone, in a story I retell in more detail in this book, we had trouble bringing some persons with Ebola virus disease into treatment centers for care because their community members were desperate that they be safe; terrified of getting the disease; and, deeply distrustful of who we might be and what we might do with their loved ones. In contrast, at home in the U.S., while many people worked to mitigate the effects of the pandemic, I frequently encountered persons and systems that ranged from avoidant to obstructive of even the most non-controversial risk management efforts (for example, more high-quality testing, integrated tracking of work and school absenteeism and influenza-like illness). Here, narratives and decisions were commonly untethered from any core wish that those people near and around them remain well. ***In short, in Sierra Leone, we faced crippling compassion, while here in the U.S., we faced a compassion***

deficit. Ultimately, the grounding in compassion in Sierra Leone allowed negotiation and healthcare delivery. In contrast, in early to mid-2020, I walked into some long-term care facilities in the center of Nebraska where half or more of the residents were dead from COVID-19. And yet, I soon afterwards sat across a table from a senior state health official being told that basic aspects of what constitutes a health risk were not science but a matter of opinion, and that people could disagree even about whether or not something that was actively killing people at scale was doing so. That person later joined as a plaintiff in a lawsuit designed to both block and discourage county officials from undertaking usual health measures relevant whether there is a pandemic or not. Despite decades of pushing our health security agendas onto others globally, we at home proved that we were just as capable as everywhere else to be another cog in the global engine fueling a pandemic: distracted, at times base, and providing a solid share of global preventable deaths.

I remain struck by some of my critically ill patients who needed anti-SARS-CoV-2 therapy, and wanted it, and yet would not consent to it because their family members and in some instances their outpatient physicians were entrenched in weirdly mixed dogmas that minimized the disease and denounced medical countermeasures, even as the patient was being intubated because they needed mechanical ventilation in order to breathe. Ironically, some of the most public-facing purveyors of such narratives were quiet recipients of the most advanced therapies at the earliest of opportunities. These populist narratives had their own transmission dynamics that were hard to predict, exacerbating their evil. I participated in a county health department outreach promoting SARS-CoV-2 vaccination at a fair run by a black church. The stall proprietors and shoppers were welcoming, but there was a common theme. Despite the vaccine's high-level of effectiveness and the realized consequences of being severely ill when having less healthcare access, there was little interest in vaccine. A man there put it like this, "If they are not taking the vaccine, why should I?" referring to the White community.

Not every step towards progress in health emergency risk management has been stalled. There have been individual champions of effective risk management, and many people who behaved courteously. We had county public health officials who spent nights in hotels under police protection triggered by real threats because they affirmed the existence of the pandemic and performed basic risk communication. Many healthcare workers in patient transport and large and small healthcare settings alike pursued aggressive clinical care at times under severe shortages of resources including personal protective equipment. UNMC and Nebraska Medicine accepted evacuees from Wuhan and later the first SARS-CoV-2 infected patients in the U.S., when little was known about the nature of the threat. My colleagues worked behind the scenes to coordinate everything from the way N95 masks can be re-used to protocols for first responder safety; and, took personal missions to promote community awareness. My research partner, Dr. Jana Broadhurst, and her team developed one of the earliest functioning U.S. tests to accurately assess patients for SARS-CoV-2 infection, enabling local assessment of patients at a time when nationally resourced tests were not yet validated nor available for reliable use, and allowing the earliest enrollments of patients into therapeutic clinical trials. She helped others develop their workstreams and assays with large impact, later designing and implementing high through-put workflows and approaches for distributed, high-fidelity saliva-based testing resilient to many of the supply shortages occurring for laboratories. This included on-site planning, training of community members who would do the collections and transport specimens, everything that then must occur in and out of the laboratory to ensure value from having received them. This helped schools, critical infrastructure, and at-risk communities in our region adopt liberal, inexpensive, and fast test-based screening. Eventually, there were analogous efforts across the U.S. As impressively, amidst pressures to do otherwise, some leaders in these communities sought and used these services for as long as political pressure would allow them to do so.

There is not space here to recount the many strong clinical and public health operators who mitigated the consequences of the COVID-19 pandemic, even if they had to do so frequently in a hostile and non-cohesive environment. Nationally, we saw early efforts to mobilize people to think about their risks and act locally. Great examples of this called COVIDACTNOW.org and COVID-LOCAL.org were convened by Professor Rebecca Katz at Georgetown University,

Jeremy Konyndyk, and several of their health security colleagues. Vaccines, biologics, and small molecules (more conventional antiviral drugs) arrived quickly thanks to existing research and development against pervasive threats like malaria and HIV. They were safe and reasonably effective, tangibly preventing deaths, though with some limitations linked to the science, public health, and product development politics that I describe in the last chapter of this book. Unfortunately, populist interdiction occurred, fueling continued transmission, new variants, worse outcomes including more preventable death.

Ultimately, managing risks from pandemics and other health emergencies and disasters is not about health. It is about us as communities of people. We either are collectively organized around cooperative aims, or we are not. We either fundamentally care about each other, or we do not. The narratives and decision making that we exercise must be anchored upon shared interests in order to be successful. As health professionals, when we conduct risk assessment, decision making, and risk communication we must insist that everyone else is part of the conversation, as well, free to focus and communicate what they value, recognize, and prioritize most. In health, we tend to seize every opportunity to increase awareness of the importance of durable investment in systems that promote general health access, resiliency, and pandemic risk management. However, we must be careful to not exploit emergencies as opportunities for health system narratives, as this distracts from timely messaging and leaves an avenue for some political leaders and others to shift focus and culpability for community wellness to constrained health systems while obstructing meaningful action. The issue for a household is not the population attack rate or case fatality rate, it is the surety that people they love and persons on which they rely remain part of how they live, and that there is recourse for the impact directly from a pandemic threat, or indirectly due to economic loss, food insecurity, and deprivation. Actions and narratives must focus on that.

What then makes people and their communities resilient and more ready? Largely, the need remains leadership; diverse, resilient, and prepared people; and, resources. Enculturation also is critical. Some of that enculturation is technical. Common ways that communicable disease is prevented and mitigated should be as understood as logging into the internet. Also, we must learn to enculturate compassion and transparency of interests. If we can do that, if we can anchor our narratives on a genuine desire that those around us are well and achieve, that would be good.

As you read or listen to *A Year of Ebola*, I hope that my telling of the daily grind of health emergency response provides a useful frame of reference as you consider your role as a responder and a human being.

Introduction

This book tells the story of my experiences with the Ebola virus throughout 2014. I am an internal medicine and infectious diseases physician with expertise in tropical public health. In ways governed by chance that I describe, I became a part of the way that clinical management and other aspects of responding to the Ebola virus disease outbreak in West Africa were built and occurred that year. Collectively, the events of 2014 was my first experience in an outbreak of what some describe as a special pathogen, or a highly-communicable or extremely dangerous infectious disease. The usual ways physicians who work in clinical care and public health as I do address the possibility that a patient has a contagious disease, try and interact with patients and communities in a safe and effective manner and practice our science were relevant to what I did in the outbreak. But, doing them in an outbreak was new to me.

I have started writing this work more than once. At first I thought that I was simply absent minded. My file transfers, failing to record the file in my cloud space, or letting my daughters' cat walk on the computer was at fault. Rather, I think that I have been acting out the reality that my flawed recollections are less relevant than the reality of what others' have and continue to suffer on the ground. There are diseases with higher mortality and others that are strikingly more durable and widespread. Something about Ebola virus disease (EVD) promotes suffering of patients, communities, those who engage in trying to research it or mitigate its outbreaks. It is a disease that brings dysfunction out of the functional. It promotes dysfunction in the already dysfunctional people who succeed on drama. No one is immune. The complex, highly resourced academic-military-industrial complex that has thrived on dedicated funding for research on viral hemorrhagic fevers such as Ebola virus, Marburg virus, Lassa Fever virus and others for years is no more or less immune than the sensibilities of well-meaning citizens in communities traveling to affected areas or unwillingly receiving those who return from them. Ebola virus disease and other viral hemorrhagic fevers are plights that bizarrely solicit more funding than the far more common cholera and even less interest in getting close to the people who suffer from it for fear of becoming infected.

Two people encouraged me to write this book. The first is a Navy historian to whom I dutifully provided an audio interview and debrief. He asked for an interview because I became known to him as one of the few military personnel who became directly involved in the outbreak response to Ebola virus disease in 2014. He seemed a very patient and bright man who meant to praise my story-telling. Instead what he implicitly said was, "You are perversely equipped to allow others into your head and this outbreak." My wife, too, thought that this was a good idea. I am not sure why. I think that she thought it would make me less angry. I think that it has helped. Mostly, it helped me to realize that most of my anger is directed at myself.

Do not believe that I honor anyone with this work. The people I know who have died from the Ebola virus ought to regard it with disdain. They would wonder whether their death reflected sacrifice and what has come of it, whether that sacrifice resulted in substantive changes in the way that the affected communities and the global community prepare for and respond to such emergencies. I am rewriting the small bit I had started near Pentecost. My church adult formation class is examining resurrection stories. We have been asked whether we see resurrection in our lives from our experiences in the events around us. I have not yet seen it from this, a birth of something useful from my experience, though perhaps that will happen. Perhaps renewed interest will occur in health systems' capacities such as those described in the International Health Regulations and apparent with common sense from the experiences in this outbreak. I am not sure that fragile areas such as West Africa have moved much in their preparedness, their capacity to respond to health emergencies since Severe Acute Respiratory Syndrome coronavirus and the advent of avian influenza A (H5N1). Perhaps after this outbreak there will be substantive health industry interest in uncommon, sporadic but devastating severe diseases like Ebola virus disease, as well as better incorporation of survivors' narratives and participation in how communities and responding agencies think about and act to ready themselves for the next health emergency. Maybe this time will be different.

The views on the 2014-5 outbreak of Ebola virus disease in West Africa by international organizations, countries, and non-governmental organizations (NGO) such as Médecins sans Frontières (MSF) are well published. Likewise, a literature has evolved around the disease and this recent outbreak of it. I will not try to recap them here. My clinical and public health views of the outbreak are a part of that literature. I cite some of them at the end of this book. My articles are nonetheless a product of having lived in the outbreak and accumulated professional and personal biases. Here, I share how the year evolved for me personally. I will focus only on my experiences across the year and perspectives relevant to the Ebola virus affected areas.

I mention some of my colleagues in this book. The temptation was strong to focus on the immense contributions that they and others have made. This, however, is an introspective book. I tried to avoid detailing stories that I think others should tell, or that I did not directly experience. Since the story revolves around my role as a clinical consultant, there are some people who were critical to the larger story of that work so I will address them.

First, readers may wish to know Drs. Tom Fletcher, Rob Fowler and Shevin Jacob. These three close friends of mine have been incredibly important to the clinical response on the ground from the World Health Organization (WHO). At the start of 2014, Tom was an Infectious Diseases registrar with the Liverpool School of Tropical Medicine (LSTM) and the British Army, serving as a consultant to the Clinical Management team at WHO, Geneva, Switzerland. His research area is viral hemorrhagic fevers. Rob is a critical care physician and clinical epidemiologist well known from the SARS-CoV and avian influenza A (H1N1) outbreaks in the early 2000s. He was on sabbatical from the University of Toronto to the same team. He and Tom created the idea of sub-specialty physicians in infectious diseases and critical care rotating as consultants at Ebola Treatment Units in the outbreak. They recruited participants from around the world and built the WHO capacity to deploy clinical expertise. Shevin is an Infectious Diseases sub-specialist affiliated with the University of Washington. He worked on severe illness management in Uganda through both an NGO and research with the Austere Environment Consortium for Improved Sepsis Outcomes (ACESO). For some time he has assisted and promoted WHO clinical training initiatives. There have been many other truly outstanding clinical and infection prevention and control deployers from WHO and NGO. One such couple is Drs. Dan Bausch and Frederique Jacqueroiz. Experienced in such outbreaks, they alternated their time in affected areas in various capacities throughout the year. Tom and Rob in particular shaped the way that I engaged and experienced this outbreak. During specific periods I worked closely with Shevin, Dan and other responders to the outbreak as well.

Second, I should disclose my other obvious sources of bias. When I engaged this outbreak, I was a WHO medical officer loaned from the U.S. Navy. I worked closely with alert and response operations in Geneva, then called Preparedness, Surveillance, and Response

Operations, a unit in the Global Capacities Alert and Response department, Health Security and Environment cluster. My role was to provide technical advice in the performance of public health work by the unit and other groups within WHO generally. I also worked on health security policy. This work often involved other elements in the organization including the clinical management team and influenza program. I have a high regard for the work of the WHO secretariat in their core roles. Many friends and a couple of mentors remain senior civil servants there. The U.S. Department of Defense's Operation United Assistance occurred after my direct involvement in West Africa. While friends of mine participated well in that operation and I had some very small roles in DoD-WHO coordination, I do not have expertise in that initiative. The views expressed in this work are my own. They do not necessarily represent those of any other person or organization.

I was deployed three times into West Africa in 2014 for the Ebola virus disease outbreak—Guinea, Sierra Leone, and Nigeria. I did not enter Liberia in 2014. Not being able to do so was a recurring theme for me in the outbreak that year.

Across my deployments, there were many recurring lessons. The reader will see five of them reinforced in the narrative that follows.

- The Ebola virus disease (EVD) outbreak in West Africa was myriad outbreaks in hundreds of communities, not a single outbreak. Each one was unique.
- Outbreaks have lifecycles. Communities and response teams experience this lifecycle in different ways and at different times. Something like the stages of grief are common: denial, anger, apathy, acceptance, vigilance, apathy, vigilance.
- Clinical care and public health are inextricably linked components of effective outbreak preparedness and response. The relationship that the response team has with an affected community stems in large part from the way in which people receive care as communities observe closely how their members are treated when vulnerable. Most of the crucial data about exposures and contacts with others is with the patient, also. The clinical care team has responsibilities to the larger effort.
- Scale is a difficult concept in planning and often underestimated in highly-infectious disease outbreaks. A case of gonorrhea in the Navy may spark contact tracing to a couple of individuals. In an Ebola outbreak, the necessary machinery may need to accommodate only a few or over a hundred high-risk contacts from a single patient.
- Details matter and often are not roundly incorporated in planning and execution in emergencies. Knowing that one thousand contacts need to be found and followed is not enough. That involves a certain number of people who must be

> found and hired, paid, trained, monitored and assessed, transported, and connected by particular sources of money and contracts built in specific ways. Simply having an expectation that two beds are set aside in every hospital for sentinel cases in an outbreak as was advocated in some at risk areas is not enough. Being able to utilize those two beds involves physicians, nurses and other staff who are experienced in their roles, regularly practiced, resourced and protected with the full range of logistics, water, sanitation and hygiene capacities necessary to perform their functions safely and effectively.

This book reveals very personal views. Probably to a fault, I am an empiricist. This is a common trait among internal medicine physicians. I know that which I observe. I am suspicious about what I suspect to be the case, even though I cannot help but suspect things about what is happening beyond what I can witness. While I may occasionally relate that which I learned through gossip, rumor and the press, I try to stay focused on what I directly observed and experienced. I invite the reader to see 2014 through my eyes.

Being at WHO

"She, in whose airless heart

We burst our veins to fill her full of hay,

Now stands apart."

-Thomas Merton in "Elegy for the Monastery Barn", *New Selected Poems of Thomas Merton*

“Going forward, we must maintain a high level of vigilance.” -WHO Director General Margaret Chan speaking on the pandemic threat of newly emerged avian influenza A(H7N9) and Middle East respiratory syndrome coronavirus (MERS-CoV) in May, 2013, at the 6th World Health Assembly

“Solving a viral mystery: Experts scramble to trace the emergence of MERS” -*New York Times*, July 1, 2013

“More than 1,400 killed in Syrian chemical weapons attack, U.S. says” -*Washington Post,* August 30, 2013

"People were—became—desperate, and that's why we are trying to fast-track the situation where national government takes over these local government functions so that order is restored." -Philippines President Aquino to *CNN*, November 12, 2013

In early 2014 I had entered my second year as a loaned WHO staff member. WHO, like all U.N. agencies, has a mix of staff. Some are directly hired into the U.N. civil service, some are assigned by the member states (seconded Member State officials like me, also various professional officer programs), some are contracted as consultants and others serve as unpaid interns for a few months. Though a U.S. Navy Commander in the Medical Corps, I was a WHO medical officer. The Chief of the Bureau of Medicine and Surgery (BUMED) had entered an agreement with WHO placing me under their control with the exception of some administrative housekeeping. I was the fourth officer to be so placed at WHO Headquarters in Geneva. For a couple of years ending in 2013, there also was an officer at the WHO Regional Office for Europe (EURO). The U.S. administrative vehicles that made these officer assignments possible collapsed at the end of 2014 because as discussed later, they were never structured in the right way. No one currently is placed there in quite the same fashion as an embedded staff member. Health and Human Services (HHS) personnel, especially staff and Public Health Service officers from the Centers for Disease Control and Prevention (CDC), continue to serve seconded throughout WHO, mostly in cooperative CDC-WHO programs.

WHO personnel comprise a secretariat for the Member States, particularly the ministries of health. Ostensibly, WHO uses seconded officials to fill specific technical gaps. In my case, as a clinically active physician scientist in infectious diseases, the role of my position was to provide in-house technical advice to alert and response activities as well as to health security policy initiatives—in some instances representing WHO with public health, academic, and other partners. In 2013, my work travel consisted of policy meetings. My work as part of the task force in response to the emergence of avian influenza A(H7N9), also known as bird flu, in China and the Middle East respiratory syndrome coronavirus (MERS-CoV) was principally at headquarters. This was true for the small roles I had with the Syrian crisis and tsunami event in the Philippines, as well. When 2014 started, WHO had not yet employed me in an outbreak affected area.

My work had been, to that point, like that done in the military on a Pentagon tour. I had spent many years avoiding the Pentagon. I entered the military in 1988 as a plebe (freshman) at the U.S. Naval Academy. In my junior year while on winter break, I took a tour of the Pentagon. At the back of a large tour group, I stood hidden, unshaven and insofar as a midshipman can be in civilian clothes (the U.S. Marine sergeant giving the tour stopped mid-sentence half way through and shouted to me, "You are in the military, aren't you?") and I looked at the rambling, long halls that stretched like web strands and decided that I would never ask to be sent there for an assignment. It looked like a place where people worked on paper documents and attended meetings, endlessly, lost in looping, cavernous hallways that did not touch the outside world. When at the end of a sea tour as a junior officer on *USS Normandy* (CG 60), self-named the Vanguard of Victory because of its role early in Operation Desert Storm against the Iraqi invasion into Kuwait, I evaded my formidable Commanding Officer's attempt to have me become a Secretary of Defense intern at the Pentagon. But this time I failed. Like most selections and assignments which I received, I was sent to Geneva because I happened to be the only officer with the requested skill set available for the assignment at the time.

There was a movement in business literature in the 1980s and 1990s to categorize companies based on analogous service culture. In my view, WHO is an Army-like organization. Like all of the U.S. armed forces, the people are good, the mission is broad and resources are limited. WHO is driven by doctrine and does not like to cede ground. And Geneva is headquarters, the policy shop. My pre-2014 experience involved the frenetic late night e-mail exchanges that all people who suffer policy perpetuate. With enough diligence, a sentence can be saved in a document. The two core capacities of the organization, convening and facilitating access, take a lot of stewardship. Like working in any large organization, I have no idea if I personally helped in achieving or sustaining health outcomes during my time at WHO. But, I hope that I averted in people around me at least as many ulcers as I caused.

WHO

The World Health Organization is the largest technical agency in the United Nations. It has nearly two hundred Member States and over one hundred fifty country offices dispersed in its six regions. WHO headquarters resides in Geneva, Switzerland. Its regions are Europe, the Americas, Africa, the Eastern Mediterranean, Western Pacific, and South-East Asia. While the Regional Office for the Americas also is the older Pan American Health Organization established in 1902, WHO formed in 1948 as a post-World War II creation. It came together as Allied Forces and the rest of the world began to focus on the tasks and challenges of reconstruction. To some degree, this explains the way that the regions were demarcated. They reflect operational theaters in the war. Much like the Centers for Disease Control and Prevention's (CDC) international anti-malaria initiatives and deployments that became part of its role in a country mobilized for World War II, WHO does not highlight these military roots. The organization was conceived in the first meeting for the formation of the U.N. The military roots exist, nonetheless.

One of my favorite teachers in science was part of that World War II to international development transition. The great, sadly deceased, Professor John Cross was a parasitology expert. For decades he was a university professor and overseas researcher, including work in South-East Asia where he was instrumental in defining the vector ecology of the long-lived and dangerous intestinal parasite *Capillaria philippinensis*—how that parasite stays in nature near Luzon and finds its way into people. Before all of that, however, he was a U.S. Navy corpsman stationed in the Pacific theater. As World War II closed, like other military medical staff around the world, he was assigned to help the nascent steps of WHO.

World War II had brought additional science and public health experts into military health systems, in some instances advancing their science. Dr. Albert Sabin, for instance, inventor of the oral, live attenuated polio vaccine, began his work as a vaccinologist while a U.S. Army physician before returning to Ohio after the war. WWII also advanced such experts from within the military. Dr. Brock Chisholm, a Canadian and prior soldier turned senior military medical officer, ultimately became the first Director-General of WHO.

That said, while I referred to WHO as having an Army-like corporate culture, it is not the Army. The Director-General carries a great amount of influence and there is a heady bureaucracy. But, its fundamental role is as a forum for the Ministers of Health of its participating Member States, in the larger context of countries' missions to the U.N. Two treaties exist ratified through WHO—the tobacco convention and the International Health Regulations. While these are important treaties for health and health security, they are not the basis of how the organization works. So, WHO does not have a built-in authority over Member State activities that is vested in treaty powers, even though these later treaties allow WHO some latitude in working in specific areas. This is contrary to how many people seem to think about WHO. WHO is much more like student council than an implementing agency such as the CDC.

WHO country offices coordinate and sometimes directly implement useful public health programming. However, their main mission is advisory to the Ministry of Health. Regional offices also are facilitative in nature. Their budget and leadership are derived in large part from the countries within that region. They have a large amount of autonomy. WHO Headquarters in Geneva is the grand stage, but it is another convening level rather than the supervisory entity of how the regions and their country offices work day-to-day. It steers overarching policy though recent reforms may re-introduce more direct control in emergencies. Over time, all of this has impacted the way that WHO is staffed. The organization does not seek the latest Professor Cross superlative technical expert, though people like him sometimes emerge in the system because they are so multi-talented, rather it needs people who can develop, focus and utilize committees, convene stakeholders on issues and organize and monitor plans of action. WHO moved from the organization that probably had many of the answers, to one designed to identify and solicit questions and answers. Its importance is convening stakeholders and experts, facilitating access that results in the movement of money, advice, direct support, policy at community, country and international levels, when appropriate. It must rely on its Member State public health agencies, academic and professional networks for technical depth.

Ebola virus

At the risk of being redundant and inferior to the information in fact sheets on Ebola virus and Ebola virus disease (EVD) available from the CDC (www.cdc.gov), WHO (www.who.int), and other agencies, or my own more focused technical literature cited at the end of this book, a few facts might be helpful for the reader here. Ebola virus is a *filovirus*. It is small for a virus and its genetic code is made of RNA. RNA mutates more easily than DNA; even saying Ebola virus is misleading as there are many Ebola viruses. There are so many different Ebola viruses that some taxonomists argue whether they all should be considered Ebola viruses. The one responsible for the Ebola virus disease outbreak in West Africa in 2014-5 is labeled Zaire, though different enough than other Zaire Ebola viruses that an early change in the molecular diagnostic test used in the outbreak was required. Zaire and Sudan are the two Ebola viruses most associated with human disease though there are others that also have infected people and caused outbreaks. Marburg virus is another *filovirus* that causes outbreaks in people. Even public health professionals confuse the clinical, epidemiologic and virologic features of Ebola and Marburg viruses.

Ebola virus was named from an outbreak near the Ebola river in 1976 in what is now the Democratic Republic of Congo. The outbreak devastated a village as well as the Belgian missionary staff who resided there, ultimately infecting more than 300 persons. Less well known is that same year saw another, similarly sized outbreak of the virus in Sudan with potential epidemiologic links to the other outbreak. These two outbreaks represent the first awareness of Ebola virus disease. The reports from both response teams are published in the same issue of the *Bulletin of the World Health Organization* (https://www.ncbi.nlm.nih.gov/pmc/issues/166751/).

Answers to basic questions about these viruses, their outbreaks, and the resulting disease have increased only modestly in the intervening fifty years. The reasons for this are varied. Outbreaks are sporadic, usually in remote places, and they sometimes end before being well identified. There are occupational risks to working with the virus that require advanced biologic safety approaches.

How the viruses persist in nature is not clear. They have been found in bats and sometimes cause outbreaks in gorillas and chimpanzees. Some outbreaks are thought to have started from exposure to ill primates, perhaps encountered while trying to use them for bush meat, food. It is possible that bats or some other vector contaminated livestock animals causing outbreaks. These mysteries involve not only Africa, but to a lesser extent Asia as the Reston Ebola virus has been involved for decades in animal research facility outbreaks associated with importation of primates from the Philippines. Once a human outbreak starts, the main manner of transmission is human-to-human. Ill persons often have diarrhea and sometimes vomiting that can spread the virus. If patients develop bleeding, that blood also has a large amount of virus. When someone has died from Ebola virus disease, in the short term the breakdown of the body makes it able to spread the virus to those who work with the body in unsafe ways. In some areas of Africa where outbreaks have occurred, ritual practices paying respect to someone who has died bring others very close to the corpse or materials from the corpse. This can spread the virus dramatically. When someone is ill in a healthcare setting where usual, modern infection, prevention, and control practices are not in force and maintained, many healthcare workers and other patients can become infected. Despite these risks, and occasional unusual transmissions through sexual contact or medical procedures, transmission occurs from direct contact with contaminated fluids or exposure to their droplets. It is not in usual circumstances an airborne threat like smallpox, measles, or tuberculosis.

Patients with the disease can survive. There are no medications licensed for directly fighting the virus. However, patients managed from the recent outbreak at modern, referral critical care facilities survived at much higher rates than had been experienced in previous outbreaks, or in this recent outbreak in other settings.

Guinea

"How many deeps, how many wicked seas
Went to befriend me with a flash of white-caps..."

-Thomas Merton in "On the Anniversary of My Baptism", *New Selected Poems of Thomas Merton*

“The Ministry of Health of Guinea has notified WHO of a rapidly evolving outbreak of Ebola virus disease in forested areas of south-eastern Guinea. As of 22 March 2014, a total of 49 cases including 29 deaths (case fatality ratio: 59%) had been reported.” *WHO Disease Outbreak News, 23 March 2014*

"What we're seeing is a pattern that's been repeated in nearly every single Ebola outbreak.” Dr. Peter Piot, scientist who discovered Ebola virus, tells Reuters for a March 25, 2014 story on the outbreak

“…this is one of the most challenging Ebola outbreaks that we have ever faced and right now we have documented cases, both in Guinea and in Liberia…this is a difficult outbreak and it is very challenging.” Dr. Keiji Fukuda, then Assistant Director General for Health Security and Environment, WHO, in an April 08, 2014 press conference

“Ebola outbreak empties hotels as West Africa borders close,” *Bloomberg*, April 11, 2014

In mid-to-late March, 2014, the Ebola Virus Disease (EVD) outbreak in West Africa was apparent in Guinea. This was the first known outbreak of Ebola virus in West Africa. Dr. Tom Fletcher, then working in the clinical management team at WHO, found me in a hallway and said, "We should go to Guinea." Yes, we should. Soon afterwards, Tom and our colleague Dr. Rob Fowler went to Conakry, the capitol of Guinea. Médecins Sans Frontières (MSF) already had begun clinical operations in Gueckedou, far to the East of the country near central Africa, close to where Guinea, Sierra Leone, and Liberia come together. The community was not welcoming either the idea that EVD was there or that MSF was part of the solution. Patients suffering with EVD can be very difficult to watch and manage. Contact with a patient's stool, vomit, and blood is an effective way to become ill with the disease. A huge amount of stigma is attached to patients, their families, and communities. The sudden emergence of a dangerous, communicable disease is difficult to understand even in educated communities experienced with cosmopolitan ideas. Sporadic EVD outbreaks are relatively rare and emerge abruptly, likely from cross-over events when the virus moves from an animal, perhaps a bat, either directly or through livestock in remote settings near forest fringes. Recall the fear during this 2014 outbreak among U.S. professionals and lay people alike with regard to healthcare workers returning from humanitarian work in West Africa. While the International Health Regulations (IHR (2005)) focus on issues around international traffic and trade, affected communities can be isolated by neighboring villages and markets. There also remain in West Africa many anti-colonial sentiments and associated mistrust.

I do not like cities anywhere in the world. I was raised in a small town carved from the Everglades. It does not matter in what country I am, I constantly try to sort how to get out of the city. In West Africa, however, people seem to like cities. Rural to urban migration is common. This, too, led Rob, Tom, and several of us to the conclusion that if EVD is in Gueckedou, it is or soon would be in Conakry.

Sadly, very quickly after Tom's arrival, he discovered that he was correct. Dead bodies quickly started accumulating at the public hospital in Donka. He worked with the staff there and soon after an MSF team arrived to begin clinical operations. Rob arrived next. They were heroic and fundamental to mitigating the outbreak in Conakry. EVD outbreaks affect communities in paradoxical ways. People avoid the hospital because they do not want to be close to Ebola virus. They also can be reticent to relinquish their own for testing and isolation. In the hospitals, regular services shut down and a cascading effect may result in lack of care for ill people from other diseases. And yet, if patients ill with Ebola virus are not isolated in a setting to receive good care quickly, interrupting chains of transmission is challenged and trust from the community is hard to build.

When Tom headed to Guinea, he informed me that he had chosen me for deployment to relieve him in a couple of weeks when he would have to return to Geneva. Other than Tom and Rob, I was not aware of other active infectious diseases or critical care physicians at WHO that would be available to travel in order to mentor the responding Guinean physicians. When Tom's and Rob's departure from Guinea became imminent, they were joined by Dr. Shevin Jacob. He came in time to be part of the peak of cases in Conakry. He arrived while Tom and Rob still were there and gradually became the only WHO clinical consultant in Conakry. Working safely in these settings requires something like a buddy system. Being alone increases risk as tasks are not shared, hazards can be overlooked, and more time might be spent in high-risk areas wearing cumbersome personal protective equipment. Fortunately, MSF staff also were in Conakry then. Dr. Dan Bausch was in Guinea for WHO at the time, working mostly in the rural eastern areas providing advice to the response team near Gueckedou where MSF was working.

With rare exception, clinical care delivery in filovirus (Ebola, Marburg viruses) outbreaks has been the providence of MSF, also known as Doctors without Borders. An amazing organization, it functions remarkably like the U.S. military health system. In the context of healthcare during emergencies, it provides a framework and logistics to deliver and accommodate clinicians of any experience in low resource settings with high levels of risk. As a professional healthcare delivery entity, it is fundamentally different from WHO or country public health agencies like the CDC. It focuses on what it considers to be the key feature of such an outbreak, the need for active case finding and isolation. MSF water and sanitation experts are highly desirable in the field. They separate risk from communities and healthcare workers. They restore confidence in local, healthcare systems that are not treating Ebola virus but focusing on critical services such as maternal and child health, trauma response and malaria control. They have an excellent reputation in the field. Care providers, coordinators, logisticians, pharmacists, contractors, geographic mappers, outbreak investigators, and epidemiologists in MSF all carry this luster with them in an outbreak response.

Perhaps because MSF has responded well in previous outbreaks in partnership with some health ministries, perhaps because of fear, MSF had held a monopoly on filovirus care delivery. With the exception of some small footprint, highly-specialized groups that engage and respond to cases while MSF deploys, other care providing non-governmental organizations (NGO) have not been involved. Occasionally there have been incursions from other actors. For instance, WHO and CDC used to deploy staff for clinical support in addition to their coordination, epidemiologic and laboratory roles. The most frequently referenced example is the outbreak in Gulu, Uganda in 2000. All sorts of organizations seemed to be involved clinically and in many other respects in the response to that outbreak. I am not sure why that was so different. Dan and Dr. Cathy Roth, a close friend and mentor of mine at WHO, need to write a comparative history of the mechanics of that outbreak and the one that started in West Africa in 2014. During the Severe Acute Respiratory Syndrome coronavirus (SARS-CoV) outbreak in 2003, WHO asked some clinicians to respond. One of those who did, Dr. Christophe Clement, a senior critical care physician from Bordeaux, France, spent much of that time locked in an isolation hospital in Vietnam. He and another talented critical care physician scientist, Dr. Francois Lamontagne from Canada, worked with me for a while in Conakry through WHO before moving on to assist the MSF site in Gueckedou. There also are examples of this in 2005 with the rise of pathogenic avian influenza A (H5N1).

Somehow, though, in the brief interceding ten to fifteen years, the idea of deploying clinicians from the technical agencies as part of the outbreak response, not just for initial investigation but in support of clinical care activities and to provide broader technical advice, has been lost from the global response consciousness. Africa is a busy place for emergencies. MSF was quite engaged in Gueckedou and not yet conducting emergency operations in Conakry when Tom and Rob began in March to insist strongly that more people were needed there on the ground. Tom arrived and immediately worked with the Donka hospital staff and started the response. When MSF was able to bring critical infrastructure and healthcare providers into the process, Tom, and then Rob, worked closely with them and made it robust with sub-specialty clinical expertise and additional connections to the public health response. All of us who followed in Conakry used the relationships that they had built. Soon afterwards, Dan was providing technical advice in the Gueckedou area. Eventually, a small number of WHO clinical consultants would be working alongside MSF staff at the treatment facility there also.

That said, those of us who were within WHO never once thought that we were meant to be the core care providers in a situation per se. WHO is not a care provisioning entity. Healthcare delivery requires administration and logistics as well as resourcing of a different sort than to that which the public health agencies are geared. One of the interesting communication problems internally in the response team was what it meant to be advising. First, there has to be someone to advise, either from the host country or as part of clinical response organizations, like MSF. Second, clinical practice works as a guild. We learn through study, observation, supervised actions, and metered, increasing independence by those being trained. There are clinical apprentices, journeymen, and masters. Advising, in particular mentoring through monitoring, assessment, and intervention, is done through modeling and participation. A clinical advisor cannot only sit in a board room away from patients and expect to successfully impact care at a bedside.

As I write this today, I finished a two-week rotation as the teaching physician on an inpatient medical service. My fellows, residents, and medical students are quite smart and capable. They do most things well without my help. But, while sometimes I am surprised by how much I can talk, I cannot reliably help them improve and pattern best practice by speaking to them occasionally in safe, sterile settings. This is true regardless of my responsibilities as the physician of record. I must walk with them on the wards and units of the hospital, enter the patient rooms, observe and participate in taking the patient's history, performing the physical examination, monitor and intervene in the procedures, go with them into the laboratory and radiography reading room, assess and adapt to how both the patients and my colleagues in training evolve over time. The EVD care setting is not different. And healthcare providers in resource limited settings are not different in these basic needs. Arguably, their needs are higher.

Tom's, Rob's, the early Donka hospital's and MSF staff's work was about initiating capability well behind the need around them—modeling and shaping how to begin to move forward and interrupt transmission of Ebola virus humanely with care that is as effective as possible. Over time, resources matured and a robust MSF-sourced Donka hospital EVD care facility was established. The WHO clinical consultants then increasingly could act in a hands-on supervisory capacity. Before I left, I asked my wife, Shelly, what she thought about this deployment. She responded that it seemed like the kind of thing that I should do as someone who had built a career in infectious diseases and was practiced working in low resource settings. We did not know what to expect and so did not have pre-conceived notions. I had managed suspected SARS and avian influenza patients as a clinical consultant. I had cared for trauma patients with multi-drug resistant bacteria infections. In these settings, I had to employ contact and droplet precautions, the same very general level of protection thought needed against Ebola virus in the field. My friend Cathy and I had a coffee together before I left Geneva. She said that whatever my expectations are, they will be proved wrong. Cathy was correct for my experience in Guinea, again in Sierra Leone, and again in Nigeria. I arrived in Conakry when that city's outbreak was mature and at the time decreasing.

After a brief stop in Dakkar, Senegal, my plane arrived nearly empty in Conakry, Guinea, late on April 19, 2014. The few people on the plane looked to be traveling for business, missionaries, and NGO employees. There was talk among passengers about the Ebola outbreak. I mostly kept to my red wine. It was an Air France flight. I spent a rather long wait (several hours) for my ride in the parking lot where the airport security was very concerned about what to do with the gringo. I never learned the Guinean term, which is interesting as I usually do. My French is challenged. When conversations in late March and early April became more serious about traveling into the outbreak, I thought that I was going to go into Liberia. By April, some of us thought that Liberia and Sierra Leone were affected or soon would be so. The Mano River area represents a high-migration zone with many tribal and familial connections. As news of increasing case counts and challenges in Gueckedou arrived, I wanted to get to Liberia to assist the search for cases and begin detailed preparedness actions. Case counts at the time of my assignment for the deployment were climbing in Conakry, however, and so I, probably reasonably, was diverted there. Personally, though, it was my strike one in getting to Liberia.

My ride eventually materialized and I arrived at the Hotel Golden Plazza on 7eme Ave. Almamya Kaloum. The management was very nice and the rooms clean and simple. Most of the WHO staff were staying there, which made coordination easier. Shevin met me and we had a brief introductory meal. We had not previously met. He was kind, patient, and very tired.

Each morning there was a response team meeting convened at the WHO country office. At the head of a long table sat the WHO representative (WR) to Guinea, a senior representative from the ministry of health (MoH) and a senior technical advisor from the WHO Regional Office for Africa (AFRO). The rest of the table was filled with technical personnel focused on various issues from the MoH, WHO, and other U.N. agencies, representatives from participating NGO and governmental missions and sometimes private stakeholders such as interested persons from the community who had experience working in health. By the time I arrived, WHO had started pulling staff from across the organization to support the response. At about the same time staff had arrived from Geneva, other regional and country offices.

Three annotations from my notebook are striking from the early days in Guinea. First, the Guinea WHO country office had the longest WiFi access code in the history of human endeavor. While they hopefully have changed it in accordance with WHO information technology policy, I will share just the number of characters: XXXXXXXXXXXXXXXXXXXXXXXXXXXXX. Clearly this was an access code designed to discourage use more than to prevent intrusion. Entering the code on a mobile device was comical. The access was incredibly slow so I do not blame them. It made even the most mundane e-exchanges with headquarters painful yet it was better than most access available in Conakry.

Second, I had two different sets of notes on French vocabulary. On the flight south I had reviewed my basic medical French. Quickly, however, I realized that I was going to have to sit in meetings as well as see patients. I really did not have the skills in French to work autonomously. I used to tell my friends in Geneva that we should hold our work meetings in French. Many of my colleagues were Francophones. While there are six official languages at headquarters, discourse is dominated by English and French as most people speak at least one of these two. All of our meetings were in English when but one Anglophone was present. I had suggested that we should hold them in French because at the time I listened only to every fifth word. I hate meetings. If we held it in French I would listen carefully to every word still understanding every fifth and my French would improve. Sadly, they were far too courteous to realize that I was serious. While on the flight I had studied the French words for pain, fever, diarrhea, bleeding; now, for the meetings I studied the words for describe, discover, should, hope, growing, team, examine. They got little use. As with Tom and Rob before me, Shevin and I would take turns going to the meetings at the country office while the other went directly to the care center. I became adept at the ten-or-so word clinical activity report. Usually, I would sit next to my WHO colleagues from Geneva who would translate for me—logistician Jose Rovira or risk communicator Marie-Agnes Heine. Friends now, they were very helpful. Not only would they articulate points for me, they would hit me when I was not following the conversation and they thought that I should say something. More outbreak-experienced than I was, that often would result in them having to explain to me why something should be said and what that might be. That would have proved quite helpful even if the meetings were in English.

Third, in addition to coordination details in Guinea, I had written what I thought was going to be important contact information for keeping in touch with Geneva. Cathy who had warned me that what I was about to experience was different than what I thought it was going to be, Paul Cox—another good friend of mine who ran the Strategic Health Operations Center and related programs and seemed to know everyone regardless of organization, my WHO chain of command, also the clinical management team, including the lead, Dr. Nahoko Shindo. My unit coordinator, Dr. Stella Chungong, was the person in the end who tasked me with deployment. The reason that this list is curious to me is that, while Cathy and Paul remained important touch stones for me throughout the year, my most steady contact from Geneva while working in Guinea and later in Sierra Leone was Rob. When Rob and Tom returned from Guinea, they immediately set to work building a deployment schedule of WHO clinical consultants. They reached out through personal and professional networks identifying and vetting infectious diseases and critical care sub-specialists who could function on the ground as participating advisors. They then built coverage schedules and coordinated with WHO's Global Outbreak Alert and Response Network (GOARN) to get people on the ground over the course of the spring and summer. Rob and Tom sat the response team meetings in Geneva on behalf of clinical management. Rob took on the additional role of keeping in touch with people in the field. He did it gently and persistently. Mobile telephone coverage was patchy in Conakry as in other sites where I later would work. Whenever I received a call, though, I could guess that it was Rob. He would let me vent, try and promote some corporate memory of clinical priorities on the ground, push a little to make sure that I was moving ahead on recommendations they had laid before their departure, and obtain enough firsthand data to advocate effectively at headquarters for clinical and sometimes broader response issues.

Clinical culture can differ from the ethos around usual field public health work. Clinicians talk constantly to patients and each other. We are paranoid about both getting things right and also not leaving problems for those who follow as we continually rotate and turnover patient care and ward responsibilities. We talk to each other before, during, and after turnovers regardless of whether we know each other well. This generally was true of the excellent epidemiologists and logisticians who were deployed to the area. For clinicians, though, much of this communication is in support of transferred authority as well as responsibility. In a hospital setting, the many multi-disciplinary processes in a hospital culminate into clinician-patient decisions and a patient outcome. We are accustomed to shepherding these processes—dependent on multi-disciplinary contributions—toward that decision point with patient outcome having primacy. While I think that this helps me in my public health work by keeping me patient-community outcome focused, it also leaves me with a perpetual sense of urgency and a self-perceived moral high ground.

In the context of support and turnovers, many of my colleagues and I ask "What would I want to know or have if coming here or working here," rather than, "What is available?" This truly frustrated my logistics friends. Only in 2014 did I hear, "You clinicians really look out for each other," said completely as a negative. Before I arrived in Conakry, Shevin repeatedly went to the logistics team to make sure that they were aware of my arrival. I waited several hours in the airport parking lot for a ride anyway. The thought was nice, though. Shortly after arrival, I started pushing travel logistics information and knowledge about setting and work for people scheduled to follow me. I sent warnings like plan to wait for a ride; local residents know that workers are coming for the outbreak, so while in the airport parking lot ensure that people claiming to be with WHO actually are (an imposter had tried to get me into a car); MasterCard is not yet accepted in Guinea which includes ATM cards; do not worry about bringing personal protective equipment (PPE) but old sphygmomanometer (blood pressure gauges) and cuffs would be welcome, ….

For me, morning team meetings at the country office were painful requirements (I hate meetings) of little risk. Despite my notes from meetings in my journal, my real work was where the patients were, where I had less time to write. A few times, though, meetings mattered. I was only variably successful in those moments. When it came to simple ideas such as, "Rob and Tom thought oxygen support was important for our patients. We need to buy oxygen," the answer was a fast yes. Who is going to deny oxygen for a sick patient? When I felt that what needed to happen was a change in process owned by other people, like any setting, that proved much more difficult.

One of my patients was an older gentleman in a large family that had several family members who became EVD patients, infected from participation in a ritual funeral practice, drinking from a cup with water used to wash a deceased family member. He was the patriarch of the family. He was slow to self-identify with symptoms. When he came to care, he minimized his symptoms and attempted a strong appearance in front of some of his grandchildren and nephews who also were patients. He was fatigued but did not look yet markedly ill.

He tested positive on a blood sample drawn elsewhere and so was brought immediately into the confirmed case area of the treatment center rather than through the suspect case area. By the second day of his care, he was increasingly fatigued, slow to respond, and was mildly ataxic—shown by an unsteady, wide-based walk. Speaking French, as I mentioned, was a challenge for me. While I later learned that he is quite well spoken in French, French probably is his third or fourth language after tribal languages. With the luxury of time as on that day we did not have many patients who needed immediate clinical interventions, I began exploring his history more closely with the help of better translation from a Guinean colleague.

The patriarch had not been ill for only a few days as we had earlier understood; he had been ill for over a week. His diarrhea had become profuse while still at home. When initially I asked if he had been drinking much water, he had said yes. Now, with the benefit of more focused translation help, it was clear that what he meant by a lot of water was a cup or so a day. Culturally, despite broad public health programming describing the importance of fluid intake in the event of severe diarrhea, particularly in children, drinking enough water was not common practice. For a week, he had voluminous diarrhea and taken only one liter of fluid. We spent time explaining what we meant by aggressively replacing volume, taking a lot of fluid. I told him that I thought that he was liters dry and that while his diarrhea persisted, he continued to need four or so liters of fluid a day on top of replacing how much he had lost. I asked him to drink four liters of oral rehydration solution (ORS, water with specialized salts) overnight. When I saw him the next morning, he had taken more than ten liters of fluid, including ORS. His interactions were faster and stronger. He stood and walked readily and more normally. It was a striking difference. The patriarch still had a complicated clinical course, but I think that he saved his own life that night.

His case reinforced a couple of ideas for me. The first was that I needed to be quite explicit about volume, precise quantities, when discussing stool, urine, and intake with these patients. The second was that when we talk to the community, especially contacts of sick patients who we know might get sick, we should provide more directed self-care instructions. Delays in care happen due to geography, recognition of illness, difficulties in obtaining transportation, and stigma, so potential patients should be equipped to handle what they already control so that they present for care less sick.

For a morning meeting at the country office, I prepared a set of notes to be read and given to contacts of EVD patients regarding what they should do if they became ill in terms of self-care. This had not yet been standard practice to do. My list started with contact the health official, seek care, drink water, preferably ORS with instructions on how to make it, drink more water and ORS, isolate where stooling, urinating and vomiting happens, wash hands frequently with soap and water, avoid direct physical contact, drink more water and ORS, seek care, avoid drugs that block platelets like aspirin and ibuprofen, and do not have sex. I vetted it among the WHO consultants, my friends in Geneva, had it translated by Francois and checked by Christophe, vetted it with the MSF team and the MoH staff working at the care center. Through Jose and Marie Agnes, I introduced it to the response team. I gave them English and French versions. I encouraged its use and incorporation in the training provided to contact tracers who identify who else might become ill from having had contact with an EVD patient. Ultimately, I would go through this same response team education and advocacy on the need for this same materiel for contacts of EVD cases in Sierra Leone and in Nigeria. I am pretty sure that these either never were used as intended or if so, only in very limited fashions. Perhaps in isolated cases it helped to improve some of the more general risk communication used in outreach to the community. When in the fall I had returned to Geneva, Dr. Simon Mardel, another WHO consultant early in the outbreak in Guinea who went to Nigeria with other sponsorship in the fall, made similar suggestions there. When I shared the same product at each location where I worked, it again was novel, and I think again not adopted. There was much to do by every team in every location and they perhaps had many tasks of higher priority. As a clinician this frustrated me. What could be a higher priority than empowering people to be less sick when they ultimately present for care? This was, nonetheless, an example of the clinical and public health cultural divide. This was not a divide that I expected. When forms were pushed to the clinical centers by the epidemiology teams, in my experience we generally tried to accommodate them. However, maybe in part because, historically, clinicians have so carefully guarded their privilege of giving care in order to reinforce a basic level of training needed to do it, when we needed something from the epidemiologists, it was not in their custom or experience to speak to communities clinically. They also may have been leery to suggest to potential patients that they should think about their care in any way other than presenting for isolation. Isolation of suspect and confirmed cases of EVD is a fundamental component to interrupting chains of transmission of the disease.

Self-care by patients was not my only windmill to charge. One morning, I received a very ill suspect patient, an older woman from an outlying village. Again, a privilege of lower-case load, which I would sorely miss a couple months later, we talked about her previous month in depth. She recently had donated whole blood in a small community clinic for just-in-time use with a young patient there, probably for trauma. Most of the places in which I had worked in the Americas and Africa did not commonly employ blood products—they simply did not have cultural familiarization and comfort with the practice. In Guinea, and later I would learn in Sierra Leone, blood product use was common, usually whole blood, incompletely typed and evaluated by U.S. standards, and often decentralized in processing and delivery to the patient. Blood is visceral, the very idea of it. The morning meeting took to this issue quickly and I believe at least on a programmatic level, transfusion as a regular practice was paused for evaluation. Ironically, I was never able to get the EVD testing laboratories where I worked interested or willing to participate in pooled blood donated screening so that maternal hemorrhage and trauma (in particular, motor vehicle accident, MVA) response could be maintained. I learned later, however, that some sites ultimately did this.

As these episodes demonstrate, my performance in effecting change through the morning meetings was quite mixed. One of my utter failures had to do with active case finding in non-EVD hospitalized settings, looking for and finding patients who might be hospitalized in other facilities and yet actually have EVD. While I was in Conakry, our case load decreased. I started with a patient census of ten to fifteen and left with a single patient remaining in the care center, in recovery. Understanding the severe case burden my predecessors had experienced and the way such outbreaks expand, knowing also by then the propensity of rural to urban movement in that sub-region, this surprised me. I believed that we were missing cases. While our Infection Prevention and Control (IPC) efforts included a training team that helped clinics and hospitals set up initial screening and triage, there was little other engagement. I sought permission to meet with the medical leadership of each of the other hospitals in Conakry. In addition to Donka hospital where our MoH-MSF-WHO partnership existed, there were private hospitals, a military hospital, and a large outreach medical activity from Morocco. I never was able to make contact with the Moroccan team, but the others treated EVD screening and risk management as a collateral duty, separate from their usual work as we probably would in a U.S. facility. Qualified people on staff with any time at all available for such issues are in short supply.

However, in Conakry, there were not existing, dedicated systems at these facilities for conducting in-house monitoring and assessment of triage and screening activities or for the active surveillance of patients already present for clinical syndromes suggestive of a communicable disease. In the U.S. this is done by IPC nurses or technicians who regularly speak with ward staff and have access to medical records. They have the authority to implement isolation precautions on such patients with hospital policies in place that assist medical teams in their response when such a suspect case is identified, regardless of the cause.

IPC is a known concept in the Guinean health system. Early in my time in Conakry, I had an interesting conversation with a senior Guinean health official after one of the morning response team meetings. He said that who they at the time considered their index case—the first EVD case about which they were aware then in Guinea—was a 2-years old child with severe diarrhea. The child was presented to a small rural clinic. The staff assessed the patient and considered cholera on the differential diagnosis. They behaved as though it were cholera, employing hygiene and barrier measures appropriate for a severe, communicable, diarrheal illness. No one in the clinic was infected with EVD.

The concept of dedicated staff, policies, and other resources for the purpose of systematic IPC programming that went so far as patient assessment, however, was not known there. I wrote a position description that could be employed as a collateral duty or by a dedicated person depending on the case load of the facility. It focused on three principal goals for each facility—exercising usual IPC practice, including in the outbreak setting, maintaining entry point and clinic screening, active case finding among patients and intervention for EVD and any other communicable disease in the hospital setting, information and best practice sharing among the hospitals with each other and the MoH. The epidemiology team was very focused and doing excellent work, fleshing the details on chains of transmission. The risk, nonetheless, persisted that an unidentified patient with EVD would find his or her way into a non-EVD medical center in Conakry, just as had happened at the beginning of the outbreak. While the epidemiology team had a large and growing data set of these transmission chains, such data always is incomplete. Omniscience is not a response team skill set. Not all cases are found. When cases are found, not all patients live to answer questions. When they do, they sometimes do not recall or are reticent to disclose with who they have had contact. This can stem from not wanting to report friends or family who might then be isolated, or not wanting to admit a frowned upon behavior that led to the contact. Even if full disclosure occurs, not all reported contacts can be found.

Initially, there was interest for this idea by the response team and the MoH personnel. If it was adopted, it was done after I left Conakry. I could not get access to the medical centers to discuss it. Finally, the

MSF site coordinator kindly brought me into a meeting with the area medical directors. Christophe joined me and did the translation.

At best, the meeting could be described as surreal. We described the problem:

- Decreasing EVD case load increases risk of delay in transmission chain identification due to delayed case finding; that is, as the outbreak becomes more sporadic again, more of the cases come from people who are not already contacts and so finding them and building the necessary data base about their exposures and contacts takes time;
- EVD has a long enough incubation period (time from when someone is exposed to when they become sick, in EVD usually one to two weeks) that someone could be admitted to the hospital for anything, even elective surgery, and show EVD while in- house;
- EVD is non-specific at its start, someone could present for care feeling quite ill but not look like an EVD patient or meet suspect case definitions through casual interview for several days;
- Responding to these challenges requires increased vigilance and specific action, helps readiness for the next outbreak by the next pathogen.

While the conversation opened gently, the responses were incredulous. Screening is performed when entering the facility. Yes, but screening at entry to the hospital only matters for people who already meet the definitions and are sick with EVD, and they might not look like that or they might come in for something tangential—a little bit sick so less aware resulting in a car accident, showing they have EVD later after the trauma surgery. But they do screening at entry. Yes, but *all* screening fails. Screening is important, but it fails, always, eventually there will be cases that are not initially detected and that could cost you many exposures. Recognizing a potentially contagious condition in a person regardless of cause is easy and easy to isolate cheaply, just distance, a corner of a room and then you call someone. But, they do screening at entry. Yes, but even if your entry screening were perfectly executed and the process had 99.99% sensitivity (it finds 9,999 of any 10,000 EVD patients, and hardly any health process in practice does even remotely that), the outbreak is still around and someone is going to end up with a case in their facility because people come to cities and come to hospitals *because* they are sick. People are not necessarily febrile all of the time when you happen to test them just because they have a febrile illness.

I was not invited again to that meeting. It was near the end of my time in Conakry. In Sierra Leone and Nigeria I again introduced this approach. I am not sure if it was adopted in those locations, either. The IPC group in Geneva when re-organized did not like my IPC management documents. The group was smart and experienced and the general idea is not possible to discount. Ultimately, it promoted something analogous. Their effort may not have been informed by mine. Processes in any bureaucracy tend to self-isolate. At the time I thought that my colleagues from Conakry must be engaging in collective denial. They already in late April-May were so fatigued by the idea of EVD that they simply were embracing the idea that Conakry, at least, was done with it. It was not the only lack of vigilance. Sadly, after I left, the outbreak in Conakry blossomed again following the usual incubation period for having missed a transmission cycle or two.

As part of this interest in increasing vigilance in testing as incidence (new cases per those at risk) dropped, I was intrigued by use of oral swabs. In previous outbreaks, swabs had been tested for the identification of Marburg virus (related to Ebola virus) among unexplained deaths. The policy for testing people for Ebola virus in Conakry was that people should be moved to the EVD care center for questioning and drawing blood for testing. In the context of someone already admitted to a hospital, though, that created several barriers. First, the medical directors did not want teams of people in personal protective equipment (PPE) coming into their hospital and removing a patient. That is probably one of the reasons that they were so dogmatic about the idea that entry screening alone was sufficient to mitigate the risk of someone being in their facility shedding the Ebola virus. Even if for an isolated exercise, practice, if the community saw that they would assume that Ebola was in the hospital. The hospital would be shunned. Second, while they might already have blood drawn in their laboratory on such patients that they could send for testing, samples have to continue to be drawn for more than 48 hours passed the onset of symptoms as early draws can be falsely negative. It takes a while for enough virus to make it into the blood for testing to find it. Drawing blood on someone in order to evaluate them for EVD means someone has to be in PPE on the ward as well as the challenge of having a sufficiently trained traveling phlebotomy team. While this could be done, as incidence fell I felt that testing should be de-centralized, distributed, less intrusive, hence my interest in the oral swabs. You can hand or even throw a swab to a patient, have the patient perform it, and then have them drop it into an open, waiting bag.

In Gueckedou, the mobile laboratory was performing Ebola virus testing on swabs for use in the oral cavity (mouth) or in blood if readily visible on the patient, in addition to the usual testing on drawn blood from ill patients. The swabs were being collected in order to assess people who died from an unknown cause so that Ebola cases would be recognized. This had started to be done in Conakry as well, but in very small numbers. Referrals for unexplained or suspicious death from Ebola virus were rare while I was there—another warning sign of lack of vigilance in the community during an outbreak. One morning shortly before I left, the EVD care team was told that an older woman had died while in the hospital and on reviewing her case file the pathology team said that she might have met the clinical case definition of a suspect EVD case. A colleague of mine, an excellent MSF infectious diseases physician, went to assess the deceased. When she returned, she said that she was highly suspicious of EVD. No sample had been drawn other than a swab. That swab tested negative. As I was curious about broadening use of the swabs, I went to discuss the test with the laboratory at our site that tested it. This laboratory was the hospital's, enhanced and supported by personnel from an outstanding referral laboratory. My colleague from that referral laboratory confirmed that the swab had tested negative. They had been receiving occasional swabs over the previous few weeks. We began discussing the test in more depth. They had not yet had a positive swab in Conakry. "I am sorry, we are in the middle of an Ebola outbreak and you have not had a positive swab since you have been doing them here?" "No." "Have you had positive controls on swabs?" "No." This alarmed me generally as the practice of obtaining blood from a vein or the heart of persons who had died suspiciously or from unknown causes had stopped before I arrived in Conakry. They were relying on swabs for identifying these cases. This alarmed me specifically in the context of this recently dead woman referred for assessment.

When I returned to the EVD care center, the MSF nurse who was handling triage calls told me that the family was insisting that the body be released so that they could act in custom for their relative. I asked that release be delayed until the response team (in the broad sense, MoH, MSF, and others) could confer. I wanted to do a blood draw for testing on the patient, if necessary by cardiocentesis, needle extraction of blood from the heart through the chest wall. I was overruled on two counts. These were not wrong, necessarily, but they certainly were frustrating in the context of my view that the vigilance posture in Conakry was far too low. First, the family was not amenable to further delays in release of the woman's body and were unlikely to appreciate the idea of violating the body by needle or knife in order to obtain sample. Second, my colleagues were by then aware of my view that our assessments of deceased persons in Conakry potentially had been flawed and that moving forward all tests on people who had died of unknown causes should include both percutaneous blood collection and use of swabs, possibly skin snip as well. The swabs simply were not validated in Conakry. Their apparent successful use in Gueckedou did not mean that it was working in Conakry. So many variables are at play from the swabs themselves, practice of collection, transport and handling, myriad test assay differences. The decision and response was that moving to a more aggressive sampling approach would decrease public confidence.

As a junior officer onboard *USS Normandy* (CG 60) in the early 1990s, one of my assignments was as the Auxiliaries Officer. In this role, most mechanical equipment that did not have to do with main propulsion systems fell under my division's responsibility. We had just undergone a shipyard period and were facing an inspection later that year by the Board of Inspection and Survey (INSURV). At that time, hearing "INSURV" was a bit like hearing the name of the

Government Accounting Office, “GAO”. It struck fear in people with and without cause for it. It did not matter how well or how long you had performed your job. The idea of being audited by a mysterious group of people from somewhere off the pier incited dread. They were not in the Adriatic Sea with us in the middle of the night when bubble gum or an unconventional spot weld seemed the best idea to keep a bearing seal intact. They cared only for how far afield the ship had been taken from its intended design and construction, whether the shipyard period had been put to sufficient use. Included under my responsibility was the Recovery, Assist, Secure and Traverse (RAST) system. The RAST system was used with helicopters. An SH-60B helicopter with a probe and line could be caught in the RAST system and helped to be lowered onto the flight deck of what was, comparatively to an aircraft carrier or large amphibious ship, a small ship. Our ship usually had two such helicopters assigned to it. In preparation for the inspection, I reached out to the aviation engineering group for our geographic area and asked for a technical assist visit. For better or worse, they provided it. The shipyard and our own maintenance efforts had done well, except that the placement of the tracks for the capture device in the system had a centimeter or so deviation from accepted ranges. The system functioned, but it was out of specification. Sorting the true importance of such deviations is hard. Maybe it would never impact flight operations, nor be noticed by the scheduled inspection team. The yard period was essentially over, however, and dealing with this would cause some ship and operational scheduling pain. For the shipyard visit, Naval Sea Systems Command

(NAVSEA) had assigned a civilian engineer to help coordinate the efforts along with the Chief Engineer. Bob Lynch was an affable, practical, and hard-working former surface warfare officer. Shortly after my Chief Petty Officer and I learned of the problem from the technical assist team, who seemed even now in retrospect a little too happy to have found an error, I went into the wardroom for a cup of coffee. Bob was there, and no one else. I described the problem. I was dreading going to talk to the chain of command knowing the impact this would have, even though I mostly appreciated that this was not something that reasonably could be traced to an avoidable error by the division. He only said, "The truth will set you free." It did, a little painfully for everyone. Bob's voice was in my head as I spoke with my response team counterparts in Conakry on this issue of Ebola virus testing of decedents. Unfortunately, Bob was not in their heads. I had a divergent view from the rest of the team on the nature of the outbreak in Conakry.

The Conakry EVD care center was a good place to become indoctrinated on special pathogen (severe, highly contagious infectious disease) case management. Tom and Rob had done the heavy lifting with MSF and other response team colleagues in establishing the site. MSF structure, function, and supply in Donka were outstanding. The MSF staff were welcoming, knowledgeable, and interested in patient outcomes. They tolerated our use of WHO supplied PPE, kept us (WHO clinical consultants) integrated in the clinician rotations, made use of us when they had questions or needed surge. The MoH physicians worked well with both MSF and us. MSF water and sanitation and logistics have storied pasts, deservedly revered. In Conakry they worked very well with our logistics personnel. Simply, it was a very well-integrated site with smart people who wanted to do good work. When Christophe and Francois arrived, once indoctrinated, they started work on improved critical care monitoring procedures, which they took with them to the MSF site in Gueckedou. My feedback later in the year from MSF staff who had been there was that they integrated in Gueckedou well, as did another friend of mine later in the summer, Dr. Billy Fischer, a critical care physician from the University of North Carolina at Chapel Hill. Like most integrations, this was personality dependent and work locally mattered.

An EVD care center is structured to accept patients for assessment and have them isolated for care and escalated for care based upon their need and their risks. In Conakry, it was a series of tents and temporary structures around an old, small hospital building. There was a well-demarcated triage area where patients could be interviewed at a safe distance by care center staff not in PPE. This screening and triage area had a second entrance through which staff in PPE could escort patients into the suspect patient area. In this area, men and women were separated as well as those who were low risk for transmitting Ebola virus (no diarrhea, vomiting, or bleeding yet) and those at higher risk already showing these signs. From the suspect area, staff could exit through a supervised decontamination and doffing lane or move into the confirmed area where patients with positive tests for the Ebola virus resided. Once in the confirmed area, staff were permitted only to exit and not to return to the suspect case area. Teams of physicians, nurses, hygienists cycled through the high-risk areas of the care center. There was a burn pit and mechanism for laundry inside the high-risk area. Sorting the timing of personnel movement through, into, and out of the high-risk area always was a trick. Delays and stacked staff waiting to don and doff PPE could occur on entry and exit. With ambient temperatures over 100^{0}F, having to wait to remove PPE represented a problem, particularly for the MSF staff who were wearing TyCHEM® impermeable suits. The WHO consultants who worked in Gueckedou also wore the MSF kit. Billy once put a thermometer in his PPE. If I remember the story correctly, in fifteen min, the temperature inside the PPE reached 140^{0}F. Unsurprisingly, this impacted dwell time in the high-risk area. Once acclimated, in the light gown and apron, light head covering and mask WHO kit, I could stay in the high-risk area for a few hours. My MSF colleagues were in excellent physical condition, though usually could dwell only fifteen to forty-five minutes depending on the day. This was fine when executing short rotations for maintaining coverage inside, executing specific interventions and moving patients. They would enter multiple times across the day. Sometimes, though, it left little flexibility for unplanned events.

One such afternoon, shortly after rounds were completed, one of my MSF colleagues brought into the suspect case area an older woman in a hypertensive crisis who met the suspect case definition. Early in severe sepsis (very sick from an infection), blood pressure can be high instead of low, particularly in a hypertensive patient who has not been able to take medications when ill. While she was able to walk the patient in from the triage area, she and the nurses had been in PPE beyond what was appropriate as a limit for that afternoon. It was hot. She alerted me and I donned my PPE while she exited. They had her well-placed in a single person tent and the nurses helped me for a couple minutes prior to their exit. Soon, I was alone in the high-risk area with this patient. While I would spend much more time alone in high-risk areas later in the year and had done so before in Conakry, I do not advise it. Staff should enter as teams in no small part because what happens can be hard to predict, being alone also extends time in PPE because things happen more slowly. My MSF colleague came to the edge of the high-risk area near where I was immediately after doffing her PPE.

The patient's blood pressure was high, 200s/120s. She was febrile and poorly responsive. My colleague got me hydralazine from the pharmacy in the low-risk area. Hydralazine drops blood pressure quickly by helping arteries relax and dilate. It was in a thick glass ampoule. While breaking the ampoule bedside, it broke badly as many of the ones in these settings do. It tore my glove and lightly cut the palm of my right hand. The patient's tent had been decontaminated since the last bleeding patient occupied it. I had changed my outer gloves—always wore two sets—and washed my gloved hands with 0.5% chlorine solution in between having accessed her peripheral IV and taking the hydralazine from my colleague. I had just taken the ampoule from the box; it had not resided in the high-risk area. Nonetheless, the event gave me a moment's pause. I discarded the broken ampoule in the container for sharp objects and opened a second ampoule. I did not want to inject glass fragments into her IV line. The second ampoule opened with less drama. She responded to the hydralazine, and I completed the intake process. In the end, she did not have Ebola virus, we think.

The suspect case area had several challenges in clinical management. In an outbreak, patients arrive ill. No one otherwise wants to be seen at or have to go into an EVD care center. Many severely ill patients are referred for assessment because higher level care facilities will not accept them unless they have a negative EVD test result. Often, they will meet the suspect case definition simply because they are severely ill. Less ill patients come as well. In them, the risk-to-benefit analysis is even more complicated as entry into the EVD care center carries unique risks. First, while the measures described do limit the possibility, EVD infection can happen inside an EVD care center. Second, the mechanics of providing safe and effective care in a special pathogens' environment like Ebola virus, particularly in low resourced settings, make doing the usual things in treating ill patients more difficult. They are less accessible to staff, seen less, have less interventions and therapies available. Consequently, I have spent a lot of time in suspect case areas with patients trying to model the care that they would have received had they been able to go directly to the specialized location their care needs demanded.

Also, I worked at each location to get discharged suspect cases, ones who tested negative for EVD from a blood polymerase chain reaction (PCR) test at least forty-eight to seventy-two hours after the start of their symptoms, on the contact monitoring list. I wanted all tested negatives followed as though they had been in contact with someone who was ill with EVD. While we took care to lower the risk of transmission from an EVD infected to an uninfected patient in the suspect case area, the risk existed. Sometimes, these patients were being followed already because they had had contact with an ill EVD patient. For them, I wanted their monitoring clock reset so that it continued to twenty-one days after discharge from the suspect case area. Sometimes, these patients did not report any such contact. For these I wanted them added to the monitoring list and checked for twenty-one days. This proved controversial at each of the sites where I worked. In Conakry, it was controversial because they considered the suspect area at this facility quite safe. I had another concern, though. I felt that people willing to risk the stigma of being assessed at the care center were different than people in the community with fever—which is common, especially in Conakry—who did not come for testing. They may have been aware of contact that they did not disclose. They may have felt sicker than they disclosed. If already a known contact, within a community of more than one ill patient, they may be aware of more contact later that they had not disclosed. Yet, adding such patients strains human resources, as such contacts have to be seen and questioned daily. The epidemiology groups variably were able to add patients discharged from suspect case areas.

The confirmed case area shared many of these challenges. Common sense actions sometimes were hard. Why could we not have a refrigerator in each of the high-risk areas in order to encourage patients to drink more ORS as it tastes better when cold? Eventually a television was placed in the confirmed case area as their stays could be for weeks. Some of the most frustrating challenges were safety issues. There never seemed to be enough blood pressure cuffs. Heads of beds could not be elevated, an important aspect of patient safety in severely ill patients because of the risk of aspiration. An MSF logistician solved that for me by making wooden wedges to raise the pillows.

Perhaps most frustratingly, there were blind zones in the high-risk area that could not be observed from the low-risk area. Fundamentally an internist, I was worried about patient-staff communication as well as falls. We had trouble getting a telephone line in place. We could not always guarantee that a less ill patient would come to the edge of the high-risk area and alert staff of a problem. There were no walkers, devices designed to help people who are unstable when they walk be more secure when they do so. When I raised this point, my MSF colleagues worked hard to get them on site but it took time.

These last two issues, visibility of the high-risk area and no walkers, I think, contributed to the only fatality I experienced among my Conakry patients. One patient died of fifteen or so EVD patients under my care in Conakry. This was a testament to the hard response work of Tom, Rob, Shevin, the MSF team, later Christophe and Francois, and willingness of the MoH physicians to meaningfully participate and willingness of all involved to embrace what I and others asked—usual care for any patient with severe sepsis and shock, regardless of setting.

That one death still troubles me. She was very ill with EVD and also had developed severe malaria. We recognized this and had started her on artesunate-based IV therapy, the standard of care anywhere for severe malaria. She was an older woman. In the middle of the night, she rose to go to the bathroom and fell. She was found either dead or near death on the next shift.

She may have died under the best of circumstances. The published data from that spring in Conakry and later case series show much higher death rates among adults in that population over forty years of age. The combination of severe EVD disease and severe malaria is an unfortunate one. We could get quite aggressive in care with IV fluid resuscitation and therapies, but we could not provide breathing support on a ventilator or dialysis. Nonetheless, I cannot help feel that had she reached extremis, had her event during the day, we would have seen earlier and perhaps intervened better. People can only be in PPE so long and so often. We were not staffed for intensive 24-hour care in the risk area. But, had the fall been observed or altered we could have entered and begun to respond even in the middle of the night. The MSF team with their MoH colleagues assured at least enough staff to alert for help every night.

Patient safety is a universal challenge in healthcare delivery. Another safety challenge emerged from an unexpected source, the site's practice of employing oral metronidazole therapy for all incoming patients. While I tended to use antimicrobial drugs in patients based on the clinical syndrome I determined that I was seeing, to a large extent that is a privilege of training and experience. When responding to health challenges with few resources, protocols are quite useful for effecting standard practice, as well as making use of less experienced healthcare providers. MSF and the military have this in common. Before I arrived in Conakry, the practice was to give an antibiotic such as ciprofloxacin or a cephalosporin for common bacterial causes of diarrhea as well as metronidazole. For the ciprofloxacin or cephalosporin, the thinking usually is, fever and diarrhea in a patient who looks sick… this could be typhoid, another bad bacteria or one of these with Ebola virus disease. If they have both, the patient probably is better with only one bad diarrheal disease and the bacterial portion of the illness should be treated. I am sympathetic to this thinking and usually do not fight it when already in a facility's protocols. Use of the metronidazole is a bit more convoluted. Some people think that with the other antibiotics it helps deal with bacteria that take advantage of an Ebola virus injured intestinal lining. The concern is that with injured intestinal epithelium, the bacteria enter the bloodstream and worsen the patient's already severe disease. Metronidazole is better than most drugs at dealing with those bacteria that function well with little to no oxygen. Those bacteria are common in the intestines. Some argue that ameba also may be present. This is possible and metronidazole would treat that.

Unfortunately, taking metronidazole, particularly orally, has its consequences. While it is an important medication, it can cause significant nausea and anorexia (loss of appetite). It also causes dysgeusia, changes the way that food and drink taste. Most of my patients who have had this report a metallic taste. In the Conakry EVD care center, I saw more than one patient experience this, though one in particular, who was doing well maintaining fluid by drinking ORS. Then, exhibiting classic metronidazole adverse effects, he stopped drinking. I then had to intervene much more aggressively. Those patients survived, but it made me very leery of the drug's systematic use in this setting. The other more usual antibiotics also had their usual safety challenges. I believe that I treated at least one moderately severe antibiotic-associated diarrhea in a recovering patient from *Clostridium difficile,* ironically in that instance requiring this time parenteral (intravenous, IV) metronidazole.

There is a derisive term for these descriptions, eminence-based medicine. These associations and observations are colored by my biases. Sadly, at the most robust EVD care center that I experienced, laboratory capacity was meager. Inside the high-risk area we had rapid malaria tests for *Plasmodium falciparum* (a malaria parasite) infection. They were not capable of detecting other potential types of malaria in West Africa, for instance *Plasmodium ovale or malariae*. Rob had coordinated with Abbot Pharmaceuticals for the provision of an iSTAT device. Used commonly in critical care units around the world for just-in-time blood gas measurements for patients who are in respiratory distress or otherwise severely ill, it generally is a useful, handheld device. Like most things that seem like they should be simple, use in the EVD care center was complicated. At first, we tried to use one of these devices in the high-risk area. It does not like operating at temperatures over 30^0C and we were in the dry season with temperatures at 40^0C. When we cooled the device, condensation developed on the electrical contacts, and it would not function reliably. Ultimately, our laboratory colleagues doing Ebola virus diagnostics allowed us to train them on the device and place it in their hot box, a box designed for use in handling infected blood such as from Ebola virus disease patients. Their space was air conditioned; they were able to use the gloves associated with the hot box and so not be pressured in a high-risk area in PPE while performing the test. They also could do so systematically. This came together as I was leaving Conakry.

Being in PPE and observing appropriate IPC practice inevitably creates challenges for performance. It is hot, cumbersome, and adds additional procedural steps to performing interventions. Over the course of the year, barbs were thrown between implementing partners about the appropriate PPE for a deployed, resource limited setting. These debates ultimately involved not just WHO and MSF but also CDC, Public Health England (PHE) and others. By the summer, one commonly used argument was that MSF had not had anyone working with them become infected. Later, there were acknowledged cases. However, an MSF-contracted local nurse in Conakry was diagnosed with EVD in April. He did well, fortunately. There were no identified secondary cases though I wondered about one other nurse who would not enter for testing. Curiously, the immediate assumption was that the nurse that was diagnosed with EVD became infected working at other facilities when not on shift with MSF, despite prohibitions in the contract for doing this. My MSF colleagues thought it impossible that he acquired the infection inside the EVD care center. While that may be the case, I have been an infectious diseases consultant long enough to have seen highly experienced clinical sub-specialists make astonishing errors in IPC practice even when donned in robust PPE in contaminated critical care rooms with organisms resistant to all known antibiotics or suspected SARS-CoV. We have touched our faces with dirty gloved hands, adjusted glasses, touched others. Certainly, an internal PPE temperature of 140^0F would have its consequences on fatigue and judgement. The nurse very well may have been infected outside the EVD care center, but it was another example of how we can cling to dogma and denial in emergencies, the potential trade-offs regarding PPE selection and the very confusing and difficult challenge of sorting how EVD care center healthcare workers become infected. Like many aspects of my time here, it was a harbinger of what I was to experience in Sierra Leone.

Focused frustrations aside, from a clinical management perspective, I left Conakry with a strong appreciation for how civil, functional partnerships between WHO, MSF, MoH, deployed laboratories can make for a positive experience for staff and patients. The work of Rob, Tom, the initial MSF team, and the Donka hospital Infectious Diseases group bore that to conclusion that spring. It proved quite useful and prescient. MSF as early as April was stretched thin. It remains an amazing organization. Its monopoly on medium to large-scale EVD outbreak response meant that it was heavily invested in Gueckedou, with multiple rotations for a heavy patient load, looking at the possibility of having to be in other countries, doing analogous work in other outbreaks such as in cholera—simply without staff to do the work. While for much of my time in Conakry I worked with two very good MSF-deployed infectious diseases sub-specialists, they were in short supply anywhere let alone in a single organization. The MSF planners made use of the WHO rotation timing to decrease physician deployment in Conakry. It became clear to me early in my time there that strategically we were in a very difficult place for clinical management execution. Before I left Geneva, several of us were suspicious that EVD was spreading in the Mano River area of which Guinea is a part. Shortly after my arrival in Guinea, I sent two related, inciting e-mails to Geneva. One was to Rob and the Alert and Response Operations folks suggesting that they start engaging the new Foreign Medical Team (FMT) initiative at WHO, which resided in another cluster. It was led by an excellent loan from Australia, Dr. Ian Norton. He was developing mechanisms for registration, norms and standards for how organized clinical groups assist in disasters to provide emergency and bridging care to victims and communities. The other one was to Ian to apologize for having done that. I hoped for early identification, training, deployment, monitoring, and assessment of FMT into the outbreak, ideally trained by and modeled after MSF operations. That work ultimately required a massive, commendable effort by Ian and others.

Sierra Leone

"Lance and thorn, and scourge and nail
Have more than made His Flesh my chronicle.
My journeys more than bite His bleeding feet."

-Thomas Merton in "The Biography", *New Selected Poems of Thomas Merton*

“This is the first time an Ebola virus disease outbreak is reported in West Africa. The outbreak seems to be slowing down, however still evolving notably in Guéckédou because the last patient was reported in isolation the 7 May 2014, which supports the possibility of a recent chain of transmission.” Conclusions in a European Centre for Disease Prevention and Control (ECDC) report dated May 14, 2014

“As of 18:00 on 29 May 2014, 34 new cases (7 confirmed, 3 probable, and 24 suspected) and one suspected death were reported from five districts. This brings the cumulative total number of clinical cases of EVD to 50….” *WHO Disease Outbreak News* first reporting cases in Sierra Leone, May 28, 2014

"The reality is clear that the epidemic is now in a second wave... And, for me, it is totally out of control." Bart Janssens, Médecins Sans Frontières (MSF) director of operations told the Associated Press, as reported in a *USA Today*, June 20, 2014

“Superstition about ebola does not help. Many do not believe the disease is real, and conspiracy theories are running wild. In Kenema, the main treatment centre in Sierra Leone, a rumour that medical staff kill patients and remove their body parts is keeping ebola patients away from hospital.” From “Ebola in West Africa: A perfect storm”, *The Economist*, July 8, 2014

My return to Geneva was an odd contrast to my time in Guinea. Many commercial airline flights to West Africa were cancelled in 2014 due to a combination of fear of Ebola and decreased interest in traveling there. My flight home was delayed. I arrived back in Geneva on May 10. I had adopted the habit of keeping a fifty Swiss Franc note when I travel so that I could walk into a taxi and get home easily. Every time I would open my wallet when on the road, I would see that cash note and think about being home with my wife and children. None of the drama that surrounded the return of healthy healthcare workers from the outbreak to the U.S. and other countries had yet occurred. That really did not start until the fall and I would never face it. My family was nonplussed with the risk. I was mindful. I would come to appreciate soon that my experience at Donka was a nearly idyllic situation for safety. Nonetheless, I had a plan to move to the guest room in the basement should I become nauseated. I used the basement bathroom. I was diligent about handwashing. The usual time before someone is exposed to the Ebola virus and becomes sick is less than two weeks. I knew by the time that the World Health Assembly, the main coming together of Member State ministers of health in Geneva each year, started that I was not going to become ill.

The first time I entered the Strategic Health Operations Center (SHOC) in Geneva following my return was mildly entertaining. Everyone in the room was in fervent discussion about something. As I walked towards the chairs around the center tables, everyone pulled to the far corner of their chairs. Apparently, even among a group of experienced public health and emergency responders, the idea of me having been working with Ebola virus disease patients and near them triggered a visceral discomfort.

The rest of May was a bit of a blur. The World Health Assembly happens each May and it is everyone's opportunity in health to push for visibility, support, and change in global health policy. Delegations from the Member States as well as specific governmental and non-governmental stakeholders swarm to Geneva. And every meeting, every event, has its own mix of utility and posturing, for both better and ill. Our technical team held a side event at the Assembly on mass gatherings. The most interesting presentation was from the Brazil delegation that had done some very innovative work preparing for health issues for upcoming events. Unfortunately, when it came time for questions, none of them focused on the Brazilian minister's interesting presentation. On the panel sat the Saudi Arabia Minister of Health. In the previous year and half, there had been a lot of international concern and attention to the Middle East respiratory syndrome coronavirus (MERS-CoV) outbreak, particularly with regards to perceived risks at the Hajj and Umrah. This was a reasonable interest, and a good example of how emerging diseases can pervade conversations even when they will not do so fruitfully. MERS-CoV has a different, insidious kind of story for someone to write, 2012 to 2015 and beyond.

Meanwhile, Guinean case counts spiked. Stella, Paul, and Pat Drury, the head of GOARN, continued to scramble from a headquarters perspective on the EVD response. Dr. Pierre Formenty, WHO's viral hemorrhagic fever specialist, worked closely with them when not in the field. There was not a lot of interest in the outbreak during the Assembly. Health has a lot of issues. Nonetheless, those of us involved in the outbreak response remained deeply suspicious that the disease was transmitting further afield in the Mano River area than Guinea. For some reason, we could not seem to get the regional or country offices, or partner agencies, particularly fussed about that idea.

In early June I went to Ottawa for a Global Health Security Initiative (GHSI) meeting. A partnership between the U.S., Canada, Mexico, France, Germany, Italy, Japan, and the United Kingdom for which the European Union participates and WHO provides technical advice. I cannot find the word *ebola* anywhere in my notes from that meeting. The resumed interest in polio was discussed. Perseverations around intercountry and interagency coordination for H7N9 and MERS-CoV as well as a variety of medium and long-term initiatives were on the agenda. The expression that bureaucracies always prepare for the previous and not the next war seemed apt. In fairness, some of these initiatives were good ideas—know in advance what must be done in order to share samples from a disease outbreak across borders quickly; develop improved vaccine stockpile management for unusual diseases;

work to make these and other initiatives applicable to any specific hazard and generally useful. No one was quite ready, though, for what happened next.

In late May, a young woman in eastern Sierra Leone was identified with EVD after a miscarriage. Long-term programming for Lassa Fever in Kenema at the government hospital made the diagnosis and surged—dropping their research work—to conduct the initial public health response of contact tracing and following. While EVD might have been in the country before then, the funeral at which this young woman became infected had exposed hundreds of people. Two foreign women, embedded in the day-to-day operations at the site and considered by the Ministry of Health to be their assets, made the initial public health response possible. Dr. Lina Moses from Tulane had built the Lassa Fever contact tracing and monitoring teams, phlebotomy teams as well as the relationships with district health officers around the country. A pathogen ecologist by training and research, she mobilized the effort that described the outbreak evolving in Kailahun district to the north of Kenema. Dr. Nadia Wauquier, a post-doctoral fellow but working with autonomy, ran the molecular diagnostics at the Metabiota portion of the laboratory, working closely also with the local Tulane laboratorian Augustine Goba. Nadia also was connected with national health assets and helped everything from obtaining PPE to coordinating ambulance collection. Lina and Nadia are no less than amazing and the response there would not have been possible without far more human suffering without them.

The Lassa Fever Program in Kenema has a storied past. Early in its development, the Tulane involvement had depth, WHO participated and physicians from as far south as Nigeria made the trip north to train in Lassa Fever clinical and public health response. I would later meet graduates of that experience in Lagos. When this EVD outbreak started, Dr. Sheik Humarr Khan led the Kenema Government Hospital Lassa Fever Program. He and his nursing team had the only isolation ward in the country. Suspect and identified cases for Lassa Fever routinely were transported there. Lassa Fever virus (an arenavirus) is a different kind of virus than Ebola virus (a filovirus). They have different modes of transmission from their animal reservoirs, we think. Lassa Fever is a recognized, seasonal threat across West Africa. The symptoms of vomiting, diarrhea, and sometimes bleeding are similar to EVD. Both can be transmitted person-to-person through contact with vomit, stool, or blood. The early Ebola virus disease patients at the Kenema hospital were handled as Lassa Fever patients, a reasonable approach if done carefully.

With the identification of Ebola virus disease in Sierra Leone, deployments from across WHO started in small scale to go there. A senior staff member from the Regional Office for Africa (AFRO) went as well as epidemiology and support staff. One such person was Dr. Mikiko Senga. A US-trained, Japanese molecular epidemiologist from the clinical management team in Geneva, Mikiko went first to Freetown then Kenema. When the response team moved from

Freetown through Kenema to Kailahun, at that point the epicenter of transmission in Sierra Leone, Mikiko remained in Kenema with Lina and Nadia. The dynamics of the outbreak there were not well understood.

At about the same time, from my perspective in Geneva, Tom magically appeared in Freetown. He had returned to the Liverpool school and his doctoral research. Unable to not be part of the solution, he went to Sierra Leone in that capacity but remained a registered consultant with the WHO clinical management team. On arrival in Freetown, in true Tom fashion, he appeared at the WHO country office, met with the WHO Representative (WR) and said, "I am here to help." Tom immediately started drafting response team organizational charts, pushing the WR to get additional workforce and assessing the situation in Freetown. He then went to Kenema. In his one to two weeks on site, he worked with the nursing staff and alone with severely ill patients in the isolation area probably much longer than he should have done, as well as providing support to a transitional care site in southern Kailahun, Daru. When he left Kenema, he had seen a rise in cases from a trickle of patients to having few available beds.

In the meantime, Humarr must have anticipated the patient census growth as he succeeded in having a large temporary structure built for thirty beds in order to more than double the capacity from the increasingly crowded main Lassa Fever ward. He also had specialized flat beds made with holes in the bottom similar in idea to cholera beds. In northern Kailahun, close to the border with Guinea and where the epicenter of the Sierra Leone outbreak was thought to be, an MSF facility started to take shape.

Rob furiously was building his deployment roster of clinical consultants. He and Tom were reaching out to every loosely related clinical network they could identify, trying to match individuals with the right mix of skills and availability to participate safely and effectively. As Tom reached the end of his time there, it became clear that no one was available to relieve him. Rob was needed desperately in Geneva both to build the deployable consultant pool and advise the response team on behalf of clinical management. I was deployed.

In the background, a subtler drama was starting to take shape with my assignment to WHO. Loans like mine are accepted on a two-year basis with options to review. I had demonstrated to my WHO colleagues that I had one and not two heads, was not rabid and might be better than a new arrival that they did not know. My assignment and that of my predecessors had been arranged with the Assistant Director General for Health Security and Environment. Dr. Keiji Fukuda, a well-known CDC alumnus who has a strong background in influenza and a set of clinical grading criteria named after him for Chronic Fatigue Syndrome, sent the U.S. Navy a letter requesting my extension for two years just before I left for Guinea. The Navy was anticipating this as my initial orders to go to Geneva did not expire at the end of two years. However, on return to Geneva and now into the summer, I learned that the Navy had not taken any action yet to respond to the WHO request. The clock was ticking on my expiration of status with the WHO and in Switzerland on October 31, 2014. Another feature that would complicate this about which I would learn later is that while WHO supported my sending regular, general activity reports to my chain of command in the Navy, Navy Medicine as an entity did not understand what I had been doing. U.S. Government involvement in the Ebola epidemic to that point had been narrow. The military had not yet been asked anything about Ebola. That combined lack of interest and understanding probably explains my friend James' success in deploying as a WHO clinical consultant in Guinea. All of this would have implications when the summer ended.

I arrived in Freetown on Saturday, June 21. Weekend mobilizations always are annoying regardless of the organization demanding it. I was staring at a wall on Sunday morning. Transportation was not available. Even if it was, no one would have been available to me at the country office or local hospitals for me to try and be of use. While as cities go I found Freetown less objectionable than others, getting to the city from the airport was comical. The U.N. diplomatic security person who collected me from the airport did not appear until I already had cleared immigration, baggage and customs. He took me to the boat dock quickly depositing me with his friend who grafted me for 40 USD over the next thirty minutes as I tried to get on a boat across the river to downtown. As an undeniably U.S. or European descent middle-aged man, I am accustomed to being a gringo in almost every culture. I felt a bit better, though, when after I had warned a field-hardened, French colleague about this weeks later, the same thing happened to him.

The hotel in Freetown was simple and clean with decent food. It was owned by an older Lebanese gentleman. Over the next few days, we got to know each other. He had come to Sierra Leone while a child and then was in his late sixties. He regaled me with stories of how the Lebanese are the great contemporary travelers, populating everywhere. He also was my guide to Sierra Leone politics, which I continue to not understand. Alliances there are like everywhere else—familial, tribal, and transitory.

After my first lesson with the proprietor that Sunday morning, I had additional ones. I sent an e-mail to the WR alerting him to my arrival. To my surprise, he replied quickly and collected me for an afternoon meeting with some U.N. interagency counterparts. The meeting was convened by the U.N. country team head of delegation, the director of the U.N. Development Programme (UNDP). The technical agency lead was WHO through the WR. The heads of the country missions for the UN Children's Fund (UNICEF), Joint United Nations Programme on HIV/AIDS (UNAIDS) and the World Food Programme (WFP) attended. To their credit, most of the conversation revolved around how to start making vehicles and drivers available for the response, challenges with identifying qualified personnel, building a UN budget for the country response and communicating more effectively with the government. Nonetheless, it was clear that everyone considered themselves experts even though none of us really were. Everyone was jockeying to be seen leading, though the WR clearly was embedded with the MoH response. The UNDP lead seemed to be grounded and have a reasonable grasp of needed steps. The other heads were most keen for a photo moment where a UN labeled aircraft arrives with supplies in plain view. Whether there would be cogent, longer-term support for the mechanics of the response after that was less clear. After a little while, some MoH officials arrived followed by the Minister. There was mostly an internal MoH debate about the need or not for mobile laboratories—clearly some there were protective of their longitudinal relationship with the Kenema program—as well as the idea of risk pay for healthcare workers.

Also on this Sunday, I tried to connect with Mikiko in Kenema. An excellent, senior PHE epidemiologist with EVD outbreak experience, Chris Lane, had joined her there. They said that Kenema was quite busy with cases, though the main attempt to start a coordinated response team had moved several hours north to Kailahun. The nurses at Kenema were facing an increasing EVD patient load. Things there were a bit chaotic. I did not know Lina and Nadia yet. While Chris' arrival had slowed the urgency of my getting there, as Mikiko had been the only WHO person on site, I felt that I needed to get there quickly. They said as much. This made the next few days very painful. I would start every morning with the WR saying that I was going to Kenema that day only to be met on the morrow with, "Why are you not in Kenema?" The smallest administrative tasks took hours… a local mobile phone, getting through the UN security requirements, finding a vehicle, coordinating supplies. My friend Jose, the WHO logistician who overlapped with me in Conakry, arrived. As I provided an increasing amount of technical advice to the WR, Jose advocated that I should remain in Freetown to help coordination there. There clearly was an expertise gap in Freetown. Shortly after my arrival in Kenema, Dr. Dan Bausch came to Sierra Leone. We overlapped again as we had in Guinea. To his chagrin, he was my solution to the WR's need for support in Freetown. I was coming to understand that the outbreak had not remained in north Kailahun to wait for the WHO team there but functionally had migrated south. MSF, understandably busy organizing its response in northern Kailahun, did not interact with Kenema. I felt as though I had to get there.

Another logistic challenge was identifying material that could be taken from the country office to Kenema. A storeroom had several cases of IV fluid bags, lactated ringers (LR). This was purchased on behalf of a public health program that did not use them before the expiration date. Personally, for high-volume IV resuscitation of EVD patients I prefer LR to normal saline as it is a bit gentler in terms of a patient's acid-base status. The fluid had been kept in a dry, air-conditioned space and was only slightly passed its expiration date. WHO rules, like most agencies', however, prevent donation of material that is expired. I simply did not know if there were preservatives or other issues that I had to worry about. Rob and I tried to get the people in Geneva who manage the WHO Model List of Essential Medicines to get the bags cleared for donation before I left for Kenema. I do not think that it ever happened.

While in Freetown I went to several meetings with the WR. He served as the Minister's co-chair for the country's response committee. One of the routine meetings was an open forum of all of the NGO. One that I attended was notable for the unidirectional conversation. Two events had put the government very ill at ease. The Minister made a very direct charge to the NGO partners to vet Ebola-related statements with the MoH. Professor Bob Garry, the Tulane principal investigator who had funded much of the Lassa Fever program in Kenema for several years from his grants, had made public statements in the international press about challenges in Sierra Leone with the outbreak. Some of his statements were perceived as inflammatory and opportunistic. The public health challenge proved real, but the lack of accuracy of the accounts and detachment from the actual response efforts were curious. He quickly became a taboo subject for the government, which threatened the important work of his colleagues in the country. At almost the same time, health information companies produced risk maps for EVD in West Africa in support of corporate clients. At this stage, the maps which the government showed me were not nuanced and marked the entire country as affected with EVD. London Mining, a large corporate entity in the country responsible for a comparatively large in country work force was considering suspending in country operations. It was not the only company considering this, but it was most emblematic of foreign investment there at the time. EVD is destabilizing enough as internal blockades, isolation and screening check points would demonstrate in Sierra Leone and other countries. The government was a bit worried about an EVD outbreak in the east as a spillover from Guinea, and seriously concerned for survival of the economy from the reaction to it. Destabilization is bad for health systems and their response to any threat, communicable or non-communicable.

I do not know Bob Garry, but I am sure that he did not intend another consequence of his remarks to the press and in the global health blogosphere. Research in Africa can be a sensitive topic. Anti-colonial sentiments remain strong. Some very bright and well-educated African professionals still believe that the Human Immunodeficiency Virus (HIV) was the result of colonial research performed in Africa. Some feel this is true about Ebola and Marburg viruses as well. Smart, well-intentioned people, especially living in different contexts, can arrive at highly disparate conclusions so I do not mock them here. I am sure that I harbor many odd ideas and I have heard ones from non-Africans. Importantly, though, these ideas have direct and indirect impacts on decision making within communities even by those who profess to know better. That the long-term efforts in country by Tulane were motivated by research got confused with their durable and emergent public health roles. The government, having this longitudinal relationship with Tulane, now was viewed as complicit in doing unwanted research. This made later conversations about the need for systematic research in the outbreak challenging. I had witnessed something similar in Guinea. An article in the *New England Journal* was published by the WHO-affiliated mobile laboratory that responded in Gueckedou along with some Guinean and international partners. They naively thought that the necessary permissions had been obtained. Because a process around the outbreak had not been established, the government there felt blindsided when local and international press made similar accusations about them. This literally halted country-level response coordination for several days in Guinea as they regrouped… no other topic became possible to discuss. This was being replayed here.

In Freetown I also was reminded of why I do not like speaking in meetings and the hazards of sitting in a public forum while wearing a WHO blue vest. At this same meeting, the Minister in the middle of her discussion with the non-governmental organization representatives present asked me a technical question about what we can say regarding movement of the outbreak. I gave a very short, equivocal answer. She then ignored what I had said, responding, "There it is, the expert has said that what I said was correct." She effectively shut down all dialog with the NGO on the point of whether basic epidemiologic and control measures were scaling up effectively. This was not a useful long-term strategy. I was reminded of a comment from a friend of mine in the Navy who said, "Nothing good comes from an interaction with a flag officer." No offense intended to my friends who are, will be, or have been admirals. Nonetheless, his warning applies to ministers as well.

Finally, on June 25, 2014, I was working in Kenema. Chris and Mikiko briefed me on the situation and introduced me to Lina, Nadia, and the district medical officer, Dr. Mohammad Vandi. He was strong and incisive. Chris, Mikiko, Lina, and Nadia worked very closely in case finding, contact tracing and monitoring and laboratory functions. Two Ministry of Health personnel worked with Chris and Mikiko managing the response database. While I was there, Nadia was supported by two PhD-trained scientists in succession from the U.S. Army Research Institute for Infectious Diseases in Fort Detrick, Maryland. Drs. Aileen O'Hearn and Matt Voorhees were very professional scientists who collaborated closely with Nadia and Augustine in meeting the diagnostics laboratory burden.

Two observations were readily apparent when I arrived. First, clinical care was not part of the conversation of the response team. They cared deeply about the patients and sought to support the care team. But they were not clinicians and had to leave the details of care support and ways the care team could support the public health response to the clinical staff who were not otherwise connected to response team activities. Second, Kenema was a quiet place with regard to health. Chris had taken the role of senior WHO-affiliated person present. He was very capable and understood the many parts necessary for effective village outbreak response. But he, Mikiko, and their MoH colleague had much to do. There was so much for them to do in their efforts to ensure that the simplest data streams were built and cogent regarding how many people were infected or at risk where. Lina and Nadia seemed to be everywhere, yet there were many district residents in the response team who really needed to have international staff mentorship. The district medical officer would be quite articulate in evening response team meetings regarding what needed to be done. There would be much head nodding. The next day, the same things would be said, the same details would be unknown, the same communities that had resisted field workers would still be closed to questions. Mohammad showed much restraint, particularly after unending late-night radio question and answer and other risk communication initiatives, attempts to help communities understand the disease, related risks, and encourage participation in disease prevention and control.

In one instance, after two or three days of successive attempts to collect an ill woman for admission to the EVD care center, several people recommended police escorts and rigid enforcement of a new national rule that made harboring EVD patients a crime. The community was isolating her and would not administer to her for fear of infection, but they did not trust the response team to care for her and so would not let them enter the community. Mohammad wisely took pause, and one or two attempts later, the woman was in care and the community was interacting with the public health responders. In medicine we often refer to this as tincture of time. Given time, most disease processes will ameliorate, or at least declare their character and guide what must be done in order to be effective. Perhaps social outbreak dynamics are similar. Regardless, Dan coined the challenge best when ultimately he arrived in Kenema and said, "Where is everybody?" Having led and assisted in many viral hemorrhagic fever responses, Dan said that usually outbreak areas were flush with international support.

The WHO response team had fought the last war, moving quickly through Kenema directly north to north Kailahun, dedicating its process to outdated information of the threat. Certainly, they were needed in north Kailahun, but the conversation moved with them and for some reason, no one was talking about the very real outbreak in Kenema, which had a catchment through the southern part of Kailahun and west to Freetown. No one, that is, except Chris and Mikiko. They were quite clear about what they had been left to address. The northern traveling troupe tried to take Chris with them. He refused. The need in Kenema was very real and growing faster than anywhere else in the country. They succeeded in getting the thin support that I as an addition could offer. But, in the end, I am not sure that Kenema ever got the help necessary for its need.

This need/resource mismatch was mirrored in the clinical sphere. While Chris was trying to make me useful in the overall response team functions, I also worked to understand the Kenema Government Hospital and Lassa Fever Program. As I have done at every clinical center where I arrived for work, I sought my local chain of command, my local host and hospital, ministry leadership. The hospital was a very quiet place. It took me hours to find any patient care activity, longer still to find persons who had purview over my clinical work at the site. When eventually I arrived at the hospital director, I was referred to the Chief Matron (head nurse) for hospital issues and Humarr for issues around patient care delivery for EVD. For the director's part, he was happy to have me work in whatever capacity, clinical or otherwise, I was willing to do once I connected with Humarr. Clearly, few patients were interested in coming to a district hospital with EVD patients. And the EVD part of what the hospital did was completely separate from the main resources of the hospital.

The Chief Matron told me that she was executing training on EVD case identification and initial management. In fact, a training course with several healthcare workers was happening but I was not allowed to enter or participate. She fully supported the work of her colleagues running the EVD wards. I was free to go engage them. No, she would not be coming with me.

To be honest, I died a little and still feel guilty at having not entered the wards on my first full day in Kenema, the 25th. I knew that once I entered the wards, I would be directing care in this setting. Not being from Sierra Leone, I felt strongly that I required a local physician's authority for work. The hospital director had been clear that authority was with Dr. Khan. We were unable to connect until June 26. I did on the first day, however, meet Sister Mbalu Fonnie. Sister Mbalu was the matron in charge in the clinical wards of the Lassa Fever Program. She was an extremely patient—at least with me—middle-aged, short, round woman with a beautiful smile when you could catch her at it. She and Alex Moigboi—a very kind, technically effective nurse anesthetist-equivalent—worked around the clock in the inpatient services, basically taking turns running the shifts on what we in the Navy would have called port and starboard watches, always either working or getting ready to work with the nursing shifts. They both are dead from Ebola.

On the 25th at the nightly meeting with the district medical officer, the EVD care center reported having 6 suspected and 26 confirmed EVD patients. The outbreak in Kenema's catchment was in full swing. On the 26th, Dr. Khan blessed my clinical work at the site, and I could proceed. Chris tortured me with a delay. Thursdays meant the district task force meeting, the general meeting of the district's political leadership and various response partners, not just the people who work in health. Chris had been representing the response team. He believed that now that I was on scene as a senior WHO staff, I could adopt that role so that he could dedicate more time to the outbreak epidemiology. In the end I would fail him as an available substitute, and he would ably represent all of us. Occasionally, I would give him a meeting respite or support. The meeting and others proved interesting. The non-health leadership was starting to develop a good understanding of the case management life cycle. Identifying cases meant not only conducting contact tracing—that is, sorting who may have been exposed and at risk of developing infection from the person who was ill through vomit, diarrhea, or blood—but also cordoning or decontaminating places where the ill person was, particularly bedrooms and toileting facilities. Safe funeral practices needed to be promoted for all deaths and specific practices adopted for known cases. Messaging about the risks of EVD had to be done in communities by all civil leadership, not just health personnel. Police had to be available but not intrusive. A district response plan had been written but awaited clearance in Freetown. That meant delays in funding. The district had relied on its usual annual budget which it already had spent in a few weeks because of the emergency. NGO present had local hires who were at risk. They had tangible resources, people and vehicles, data entry people, who could matter to the response. The tenor was altogether different from being in the capital. Both the threat and the response were very real to them. They had all of the prescience and none of the money.

Several controversial issues were raised at the meeting. Curfews were considered. A "snitch line" was discussed, where anonymous reporting of ill persons could occur. A rule was established to conduct screening of all persons across district lines, in particular from Kailahun and Kenema districts. They discussed doing the same on the international borders along Kenema district. We had a long talk about the implications of international trade and traffic disruption relevant to the way that the International Health Regulations attempt to govern how countries behave with each other with regards to a communicable disease threat, how those actions ought to be considered only in conjunction with the national government. They asked for advice on blood donation practices. We echoed some of the conversations in Conakry. This group was very well-versed in the concomitant challenge of maternal hemorrhage in pregnancy in their district as well as trauma. In the end, the district complied with the domestic, across district screening rules, did not autonomously block international borders and suspended blood donations.

After the meeting, I went to the EVD care center. It was located inside the KGH compound. KGH was bordered at the back by a neighborhood, on one side a mosque, the other a field and along the front by a commercial street. The main entrance had a gate, though it was possible to enter the compound by the yard in front of the mosque without obstruction. An ambulance entering the compound through the main gate would face the main ambulatory portion of KGH, turn left to a parking area large enough for turning around in front of a small building which had a foyer, small equipment room and 4 patient rooms. This ten-bed setup was being used as a suspect case ward. Its small front overhang was where Lina's phlebotomy team registered the patients, took an initial history completing the case investigation form, and collected a blood sample. Further to the left of that driveway was an interior gate. Beyond it was the original Lassa Fever program ward. It had a couple of trailers for offices and supplies, a small supply room, and a nurses' station separated from the inpatient area by chicken wire, rusted, broken chicken wire with a sharp fringed handover portal. This building had twenty-eight beds being used for confirmed patients. Both the suspect case building and the Lassa Fever ward buildings were concrete with poor lighting and plumbing, generally in poor repair and supply. Most of the mattresses were bare. There were no bed linens and fewer mosquito nets. An ambulance could drive alongside the Lassa Fever ward and empty a patient, ostensibly be decontaminated and return back through the gates to service. Healthcare workers entered the inpatient ward through an outside door in front of the nurses' station. They exited by walking through a common area used by both patients for washing and hygiene staff doing laundry though who were not wearing PPE. There were showers and toilets there. The area for doffing PPE and decontamination was not manned reliably nor did it reliably have chlorine solution for spraying persons or washing hands. Just beyond that area was a large, temporary structure. It had a twenty-six bed inpatient area connected to the common area behind the Lassa Fever ward by a covered walk, and a large nurses' preparatory area accessible from the other side of the driveway ostensibly by people remaining at low risk. Further along that path were temporary barriers which demarcated a common, outside area for patients in that structure. On the other side of those barriers, now also behind the suspect case ward, were the laboratory and Lassa Fever program offices where the response team was based.

It was a complete, deadly mess.

I could describe the patient and staff flow ten more times with no more clarity because no reasonably experienced EVD outbreak response professional would design things this way. These capacities accumulated over time. The staff was too overwhelmed by growing need to effect change. I raged against the basic design and flow, begged for fences and walls to be opened and moved, and other interventions to make things happen and move logically and safely. I am sure that Tom before me did the same, perhaps exactly the same things. I know that those who followed us later did similar things. Eventually, after I had left, external clinical staff were there with enough density and ultimately with local logistics support that they were able to effect some changes. No number of walk-through events with the Chief Matron and program people and pleading seemed to make a difference for me. I was utterly ineffective in making footprint changes. I was only marginally effective at making process and staff work changes.

As any quick read of MSF or WHO guidance will inform, in a special pathogens unit, a place where care of patients happens where there is a high communicable disease risk, unidirectional flow is important. It is essential for safe and effective practice not only that staff are present in sufficient numbers and with training which enables them to practice care minimizing fatigue, maximizing performance and safety, and that there are sufficient water and sanitation and hygiene resources present to allow work to be in an efficient and secure environment, but as a matter of doctrine, people and supplies move from low-risk to increasing risk, ultimately to monitored doffing (removing) of PPE and decontamination before returning to low-risk. It is what ought to be intuitive for people placing themselves and their ability to care for patients at risk but often is not. Admittedly, I had the advantage of being taught these things in an established footprint that provided such care in Conakry.

When I arrived in Kenema, Metabiota had been supplying PPE for the compound for several days. They stocked Tyvek coveralls, gloves and masks. This was different from the much lighter WHO provisioned PPE which I used in Conakry. Fortunately the weather in Kenema was a bit cooler than Conakry, though still very humid with highs occasionally near 100^0F. The entry station at the inpatient ward, however, was scant with PPE despite the initial ready supply. Staff often was using washed cloth PPE or making improvisations. Worse, handwashing stations inside the ward and in the doffing/ decontamination area were not supplied with chlorine solution. None of the hygiene staff was monitoring the exit of personnel or assisting. Basic medical supplies on the ward were scant. I would spend a lot of time over the coming weeks trying to reinforce basic supply and execution, monitoring and assistance in the doffing/ decontamination area and principles of staff and patient flow. While processes would be a bit better when I was present, I am sure that they were lapsed overnight and during periods of the day when I had to be elsewhere. I lost count while in Kenema of the number of times I doffed PPE after several hours of rounds with close contact with dozens of patients without chlorine solution, alone and sometimes in the dark. I adopted pre-flight checks before entering the ward. This would prove helpful later in Lagos. Before each entry into the ward, I would sweep through the donning and doffing areas ensuring that appropriate supplies were on hand and that chlorine solution was mixed and staged for my exit.

This would not always prevent a problem when I exited, but it at least decreased the frequency of surprises.

On my first day on the wards, there seemed to be a fair number of nurses available. They reported running three shifts: 8am to 2pm with fourteen nurses, 2pm to 8pm with ten nurses, and 8pm to 8am with six nurses. The census count I had heard the night before seemed light to the reality. Several beds were positioned in the hallway of the Lassa Fever (old) ward.

The next day, Friday, June 27, I adopted a practice Tom had suggested from his experience there. After my morning rounds caring for patients in Kenema, a WHO driver took me a couple hours north to Daru in southern Kailahun district to the site of a transitional care unit. Led by two clinic officers, Ibrahim and Alpha, as well as four nurses and a laboratory technician, the unit acted as a triage and holding area for suspect cases, initiating care and facilitating transfer to either Kenema or Kailahun once a case was confirmed. At their request, most patients from Daru came to KGH. There were natural family ties in southern Kailahun with Kenema. Also, mining companies had contracted the construction of good roads that covered most of the trip. Even though Kailahun and the newly opened MSF facility (they opened with thirty-two beds on June 24) were closer geographically, the drive to KGH was faster and easier.

Ibrahim was very proactive. He often would ride with local ambulances and interface with tribal chiefs in order to assist case finding. Sometimes he would have few suspect case patients. At other times, he would have fifteen to twenty patients. Despite occasionally being overwhelmed, the staff at Daru was well organized. They had received MSF assistance in lay-out and developing IPC processes for general staff and patient flow from the outset. While there were a few issues in their flow, particularly with heavier patient loads, as well as practices with patients that we still had to work through, their situation was markedly better than KGH. I remained in close contact with Ibrahim during my time there, as did Lina and Nadia. I made trips to support him, particularly with the sicker patients, as often as I could when able to make time away from KGH. But KGH was about to become a more difficult situation.

At the end of a morning rounds in Kenema, I was at the nurses' station when a heated discussion began outside. I walked over to Sister Mbalu to see if I could assist. She was speaking with several people from the community. Once she saw me, she immediately stopped talking, came toward me, and pushed me inside. Having the middle-aged white man who does not know anything about Kenema in the conversation was not going to be useful. Several from among the locals in the compound people had joined the conversation. It became increasingly hostile and then migrated further away. By the time I returned from Daru to KGH, we had difficulty re-entering the compound of the hospital. It had become very quiet, then became very noisy. A large crowd of people collected at the front gate and began attempting entry, screaming and throwing rocks. An ambulance in another part of the catchment area had been stopped and burned. Fortunately, no one was hurt. Apparently, family members from one of the patients in the EVD care center had been informed by a third party that the patient had died. They were extremely angry and wanted to perform a funeral rite. The patient was alive but too ill to come to a common area and interact across a safe distance with the family. In a well-controlled field clinical setting, had I understood the disagreement earlier, I would have invited senior members of the group to come visit the patient with guidance while in PPE. Eventually, the unrest stopped for the evening, probably for Friday evening prayers at the mosque. Saturday was a scheduled mandatory home cleaning day in Kenema enforced by police. That and it being the weekend contributed to preventing further unrest at the gates that weekend. This was a preventable misunderstanding that more clinical resources, record keeping, and onsite care center risk communication support could have prevented. It had some durable consequences.

By Saturday, June 28, the EVD care center at KGH had three suspected and forty-two confirmed EVD patients. A combination of the weekend, the unrest, and harassment of healthcare workers in the community while commuting into the hospital resulted in only two people attending to patients in the high-risk area over the next few days, Alex and me. The next day Dan arrived in Freetown. It would take several days for logistics to align to bring him to Kenema. I then sabotaged his arrival further. I am pretty sure that he has not yet forgiven me for it. In my mind the rapid rise of case counts coupled with at least pockets of local dissatisfaction and resistance in Kenema meant that Freetown would soon see patients as ill people fled west despite the new district crossing screening measures. The WR and MoH were in desperate need of senior technical advice so that they could improve the response and prepare for more cases. And, much like the international foreign medical team gap which I still hoped would be filled, a durable solution in Kenema required mobilization of the national healthcare services with training and rotation into the area. Dan took that challenge and worked in Freetown over the next week.

Unfortunately, the case load at KGH continued to rise and began to do so more rapidly. We quickly had a census of over eighty patients with variable staff support. Efforts launched in my first couple days to use protocols for aggressive volume and electrolyte replacement in ill EVD patients with diarrhea, routine anti-malarial treatment in the absence of readily available malaria testing, and other measures became sporadically useful in the absence of staff. Some days I was alone, on others Alex—sometimes with help—would be with me and maintaining care between my entries. This was a very dangerous period for the staff.

For the most part during this period we were relying on the Lassa Fever-experienced nurses. The assumption was that their experiences handling another communicable viral hemorrhagic fever was easily translatable to managing the risks from Ebola virus disease. Perhaps they are. But Lassa Fever virus outbreaks in Kenema had been smaller with fewer very sick patients with high volume diarrhea and so their usual IPC and other patient management processes were more stressed under EVD. EVD may have a higher attack and case fatality rate… more people may be innocuously infected and survive Lassa Fever virus infection. When I arrived, there were a few Lassa Fever program nurses either in or who soon entered care as patients in the ward. They were infected early in the outbreak. This could have occurred before the current outbreak in Sierra Leone was recognized or before the number of patients presenting to the program who actually had EVD was understood. This period with high patient load and few staff created another wave of infected healthcare workers and several deaths.

Why individual healthcare workers, particularly in an EVD care center, become infected is hard to ascertain. As with the Conakry MSF-contracted nurse who developed the disease, cause is elusive and could come from work, extracurricular activities, being a part of the community. There remained a small trickle of cases from among the Lassa Fever program and other EVD care center staff across the outbreak. But there were these two waves. Given the timing of their symptoms, Alex and Sister Mbalu almost certainly were infected in that week. I wanted to stop their exposure risk and even close KGH, but this was their community with EVD and they were going to support the patients that came for care regardless of what anyone said or tried to do to intervene. The patients had to go somewhere. They had adopted the ethics of conjoined risk with the members of their community, particularly their co-workers.

During this time, I tried to solicit help from MSF in Freetown and Kailahun. Connectivity was poor; they were overwhelmed in their own ways. Ian was working furiously to get other FMT involved but none yet had committed to participating. One day I was in the suspect case ward and the MSF ambulance arrived from Kailahun. They must have come south for supplies and decided to stop by KGH for reasons I do not know. A woman emerged from the back of the ambulance, and I thought that she might be the MSF coordinator for the Kailahun

EVD care center which is MSF operated. I had heard that she was experienced but had not been able to reach her. I stepped forward, still inside, in my PPE and tried to engage her from a safe distance, to see if she would wait to talk until I could doff PPE. I know how the scene looked. We had patients everywhere, and I was operating out of necessity in completely unacceptable ways for a properly done EVD care center. There were very few people working. She left and I do not blame her, though I would have really appreciated a couple days with her logistician and water and sanitation person. They must have come to Kenema a few times for supplies from Kailahun. However, I never saw them at Kenema again. The little impact I had could not survive an overnight trip by me to north Kailahun and back.

In contrast to my experience in Conakry, the WHO and MSF relationship in Sierra Leone was at best detached and at worst antagonistic. Later in Freetown, just before exiting the country, I had a helpful conversation with the MSF country coordinator regarding consultation for a MoH facility planned at Lakka. I think in Kailahun MSF thought that WHO was trying to manage KGH as a WHO EVD care center, perhaps feeling indignant and even threatened. This could not be further from the truth. Sierra Leone was running an EVD care center at its long-term programming in Kenema. I and others from WHO started simply trying to support the Sierra Leone staff in their management of their own program by what we hoped would be helping them to refine their practice of care. Faced with the reality of the situation on arrival, I immediately started looking for actual health service providers (not public health agencies) that had the appropriate staffing, logistics, and water and sanitation support to step into the astonishing level of need. No one came. Advising is difficult when there is no one to advise. I would not have minded a conversation with MSF about how to divert all patients to their facility. For the KGH EVD patient population, though, theirs was too small and not well placed. Even with their thirty-odd bed capacity they had to spend a significant amount of time closed to admissions and had their own local challenges. There was no good solution for Kenema then.

One of the more difficult challenges of working in Kenema was sometimes having to be away from the high-risk area. Kenema was a little cooler than Conakry. Though wearing Tyvek coveralls and apron, I was able to stay longer in the high-risk area, in some instances four or more hours. Eventually, I had to leave, particularly when spending a significant amount of time alone inside. Sometimes I was well accompanied in the high-risk area by nursing staff. During the worst periods of staffing, when inside I might be the only person anywhere in the high-risk area with more than eighty patients. Even Alex had to rest occasionally. I would place or remove peripheral IV lines, distribute ORS packages, mixing or tasking others to mix the solution, change IV bags I had prepped with electrolytes before entering, pick people up from the floor, clean, administer pain medication when available, try and interact with people. I am extremely lucky to not have become infected. No one should be doing procedures alone in a special pathogen high-risk area as having someone present to observe for incorrect practice, assist in execution, and aid in an emergency is critical to safe practice. Rationally, I know that I should have spent less time inside the high-risk area across the outbreak, especially in unconstrained situations. I cannot help but feel that I did not spend nearly enough time in PPE.

After morning rounds, I usually would go to the small room used as a coordination office and library by the outbreak response team. It was one of the few spaces with a working air conditioner. I would sit and try and replete water and offload heat before getting a little bit to eat and rounding in the afternoon. I felt ridiculous, sitting there while Chris, Mikiko, and Lina scrambled with myriad tasks. They had so much on their plates. Once someone made a joke about needing to find me work to do, another time about my lunch-time life of leisure. I wanted to find a quiet place to vomit.

Often after a few minutes of trying to shed heat, I would make rounds to the district storeroom to inventory and request supplies. The KGH pharmacy and storeroom would not supply us. There was a long history of politics in the air always between the Lassa Fever program and the hospital. I would try periodically to engage the obstetrician and her service in ensuring that they were using standard precautions as sometimes EVD patients, like Lassa Fever virus patients, present with maternal hemorrhage. There was a European Union-funded ophthalmology center that I briefed. I tried to get the police and military medical systems to participate in surveillance and case referral as well as manning support of the EVD care center. These healthcare points were variably active at best. While we had great difficulty getting staff to come to the EVD care center, we had more success with the KGH screening for all persons entering the compound. Chris worked a lot with them on procedures and also provided information assessing how well the handheld thermal scanners worked in that population. The answer is, it depends.

Once during my break between rounds, Lina, Mikiko, and I made a quick drive to Bo, the district immediately west of Kenema. There were suspect cases coming from that district to Kenema. They, like all districts, were supposed to have a limited suspect case holding capacity. As we could not vouch for the safety of patients in Kenema, we wanted to assist them in standing that capacity and encourage them to use it. Also, Lina and Mikiko had data collection and transfer questions for them about the cases that they might be seeing. The Bo district hospital looked a lot like KGH only there was routine healthcare business happening. Staff from an MSF hospital in the southern part of the district had come to it and helped them set up a small two to five bed ward for suspect case patients. It was staffed by two nurses and a collateral duty physician with other responsibilities in the hospital. It had not been used. Bo had at that point three confirmed cases that passed through KGH. District public health personnel were following twenty-one contacts with sixty volunteers for contact tracing and monitoring. However, the district medical officer was quite clear. Despite their capacities, they were going to send all of their cases under investigation, all of their suspect case patients to Kenema.

In addition to the public health and clinical care dramas, there were administrative challenges. The immediate movement of the bulk of the field WHO team in Sierra Leone north to Kailahun had a variety of support challenges. Vehicles and staff sometimes would pass through Kenema north to the Kailahun footprint without any layover to deliver supplies. Chris, Mikiko, and I were an operational anomaly for them despite our increasingly higher contact and case burdens. Remarkably, despite positioning in the capitol to be seen providing support by the UN interagency, the remainder of the UN team had even less interaction with eastern Sierra Leone. At the time of the riot early during our stay, when the hospital was locked down behind gates and ambulances burned, we had no useful contact. At the height of those issues, out of concern for the Kailahun group whose situation I did not fully understand yet, I attempted to connect to support through the U.N. Diplomatic Security Service (UNDSS) country office. My concerns were dismissed by the night team and contact with their leadership refused. I had better connectivity with my friends in Geneva (I had called Paul and Rob) than I did with in country UNDSS support. Ultimately, we got much improved services including interfacing with the local police for staff movement as well as regular visits by the country office and sub-regional personnel. Dr. Keiji Fukuda, Assistant Director General for Health Security and

Environment, had intervened from Geneva to improve staff safety on the ground.

Political issues at the local level continued, particularly on the subject of checkpoint screening. Officials used district border screening for EVD both as a deterrent to travel due to long lines as well as a mechanism to capture fleeing cases. Domestic border screening is not well studied in Ebola virus disease control. While many of us worry that benefits from the occasional identification of a symptomatic case do not outweigh the harm of disruption of services, economic traffic disruption and lost wages, stigma from such practice, checkpoints along Kenema's district borders identified at least a few cases while I was there. Finding these cases is a self-reinforcing phenomenon for decision makers. These checkpoints were security operations with medicalized screening tents. Heavily armed police and military units enforced the stops. Government healthcare staff populated the screening stations. I was envious of the number of staff that each checkpoint had. I would have loved to have those personnel in the EVD care center. That kind of staffing would be more effective and safer once trained. The screeners at these checkpoints also seemed to be well stocked with PPE, heavily garbed in WHO style PPE with frequent changes each shift. I marveled at this, especially as often the EVD care center relied on poaching the diagnostic laboratory's stock. Ironically, these screening checkpoints required very little PPE. Even if a patient is ill with EVD and vomiting, simply taking a three-foot distance from the patient and the vomit is protective and sufficient for most of the interaction.

At first, local officials sought WHO participation at the checkpoints. I was leery of the message that blue WHO vests and T-shirts might send in these population level isolation measures. Our main interest overall was voluntary community participation in case finding and treatment, contact identification and monitoring. Next, local officials sought WHO and other UN staff participation as subjects in the screening process each time an official U.N. vehicle crossed a district border. Entire day and even overnight delays, where travelers awaiting screening were held at checkpoints until the following day when screening personnel returned, were commonplace. In my case, I was alone as a clinician much of my time in Kenema. I could not support Kenema and Daru, as well as occasional public health outreach in Bo, under such circumstances. For cross-border contact tracing and monitoring teams, as well as child feeding and other critical health programs, this was problematic. Also, West Africa has a troubled past. U.N. staff have diplomatic immunity and guard it everywhere for a reason. It had been ten years since the area suffered a civil war. Those memories were long, however, and many pretenses can be applied in conflict to disrupt international humanitarian efforts. Some in the outbreak referred to the Mano River region with the affected countries as politically fragile. I, at least, was not willing to start the slippery slope of allowing other "blue" vehicles to be stopped with this pretense by becoming complicit in an unnecessary intervention contrary to diplomatic custom and more importantly health response exigencies. On the other hand, I think that most of these checkpoint personnel simply were trying to respond to an emergency with the orders that they were given. Police and military personnel often did not understand why—or at least did not agree that—emergency health responders should be treated differently as they crossed checkpoints. Exceptions make bad examples. After all, they were stuck enforcing movement restrictions at the checkpoints rather than attending to other work or their personal lives. They also know that U.N., U.N. marked, or NGO vehicles might be operated also in non-emergency capacities, or by others who have nothing to do with the emergency response and abuse the privileges.

In some instances, the interactions became quite tense. I would come back towards Kenema from visiting Daru, fatigued from morning rounds in Kenema as well as the work with Ibrahim and Alpha, hungry and very anxious to get back on the Kenema wards or at least to check in with the nursing staff, if they were present. It did not help that I also was a senior military officer with strong biases regarding appropriate weapons discipline, subordination of security services to civil authority, and citizen autonomy. In short, I was an ass in those situations and quite lucky that the Sierra Leone security personnel at site generally were more patient than I. It also helped that Chris had dragged me and, more importantly, continued himself to attend important district leadership meetings. In each case I was stopped, challenged, instructed and cajoled, assessed by onsite chain of command, and finally allowed to pass, thanks to a telephone call to district police leadership.

The most pronounced dramas, though, were the dramas on the wards.

One of the most important concepts that I tried to instill everywhere I worked was the basic idea that before entering a high-risk area, staff should be prepared in such a way that they maximize time with the patient and minimize their risk. The classic example of this is in the administration of intravenous (IV) fluids, electrolytes and medications. Instead of donning PPE and entering the high-risk area, then at the bedside preparing equipment, opening needles, breaking vials, mixing components and then approaching the patient, do everything possible in the low-risk area. Enter the high-risk area and prepare the flow of the procedure at the bedside by placing prepared items, sharps containers and other safety equipment, practicing the steps while talking with the patient and then perform the needed task. I, like my colleagues throughout the outbreak, advocated that any vials that needed to be broken could be done in advance. Needles to place potassium into containers of IV ringers lactate solution, for instance, could be done in low-risk areas, resulting in one less needle, one less step, a few less minutes not focused on patients when in the high-risk area.

A critical step to achieving this kind of habit is proper staging in the low-risk area of the necessary supplies. Sufficiently stocked supply and preparation rooms go a long way to reinforce a systematic approach to being better prepared when entering a high-risk area. After failed negotiations with the hospital storeroom but successful coordination with the district supply office, I finally was able to get a reasonable collection of supplies released for the EVD ward. The next day, after having reviewed the plan several times with my local colleagues, I walked expectantly into the nurses' station before rounds in order to guide them through pre-entry preparations. As I stood on the stairs to enter that room, I saw Alex and asked if the supplies were inside for the preparations. He asked me to wait a moment as he walked past me towards the decontamination area without PPE. I stopped him. "Where are you going?" He was going to get the supplies. The container that had been used for routine supplies was inside the high-risk area, immediately next to where patients showered, visited an outside latrine and washed clothes from a broken waterspout. Last night they had moved, without PPE, all of the hard-won supplies into the high-risk area, because that is where they always kept supplies. I was astounded. Despite all of the discussion and direct supervision, the plan was derailed. I had made a classic gringo mistake. In Sierra Leone the most common word for white man that I heard—I had to ask, everyone I met was too polite to offer it without a lot of prompting—was *poi-boiy*. That is my own transliteration. The internet has failed me in finding a better one. I failed, although I had worked in poorly resourced areas for years; knew that there was an understanding gap; knew that my local counterparts had routine practices that had become ingrained and were linked to their own likely rational notions; had asked specifically about the details of what would happen; knew that my counterparts were better linguists than me and spoke English quite well probably as their third language so inevitably would have subtle challenges. Knowledge alone had not helped me.

While many people who have not worked with Ebola virus tend to think of EVD patients as terminally ill, the patients in Kenema could be quite ill or in recovery. My clinical observations in Guinea were reinforced. Coached intake of oral rehydration solution was often my best tool. Less ill patients on the wards often helped to ensure that sicker patients who could respond took more fluid. Pre-entry preparation was all the more critical as I daily would spend hours in PPE simply doing attendant tasks, placing, removing, or maintaining peripheral IV lines, cleaning, collecting confused patients from the floor. The hardest patients to manage were those with severe diarrhea, those older patients with cognitive changes, and pregnant women. Hiccups, in some patients, seemed to be a correctable sign of getting behind in replacing a patient's volume with fluids. Patients who had small joint pain either on arrival or during recovery did better, suggestive of an immune complex joint syndrome like I had seen in children in the U.S. recovering from meningitis. Clearance of viral markers from the blood by molecular testing such as polymerase chain reaction (PCR) could take days to weeks in a clinically recovered patient. Young patients could decompensate and die quickly. Patients seeming to recover slowly with decreasing viral loads by PCR could suddenly worsen with signs of severe disease, high viral loads and die. Coinfection with malaria, HIV, tuberculosis, or other infectious diseases as well as complications of underlying disease were common including nutritional deficits. I became frantic for the provision of Plumpy Nut®, a common developing-world supplement for children with severe malnutrition provided through UNICEF, and when able multivitamins.

Basic provision of food and water were challenging. Getting the money together, having the food and water delivered, having it brought to a place where patients could reach it were constant challenges, especially during periods when no staff came to the hospital.

In Kenema I had my first experiences with pregnant EVD patients. While there have been a couple of isolated cases by others talking about survival of the fetus, all of my pregnant patients lost their unborn children. When we admitted a pregnant patient, I would spend time with the shifts when staff were present bracing them for the potential shock of spontaneous abortion and bleeding. We would be aggressive giving fluids. While blood services were patchy, we would try and transfuse in advance of fetal loss. We would have antibiotics ready that are used when people had retained fetal products. I tried several times to engage the obstetrics group to see if I could get their help in sorting safe dilatation and curettage in this setting, also to discuss their general IPC practice in their setting. I was not successful in getting them interested in working with us, however. To their credit, though, obstetrics services remained available for presumably non-EVD infected women through most of my time in Kenema. Some of the expectant EVD-infected mothers survived, some did not. They seemed to die at a higher rate than my other patients. The best success we had was in not having the staff and patients near them afraid of what was going to happen, but rather partner in making the patient as comfortable and supported as possible.

When I arrived in Kenema, Humarr—Dr. Khan—was difficult to find. He had many roles—head of the Lassa Fever Program at Kenema, advisor to the Ministry of Health for dangerous pathogens, local private physician. His first endorsement of my work was by telephone. Ultimately, during my time there he rounded a couple of times with me. Both times that I know he rounded without me would later haunt me for drastically different reasons.

When Humarr and I first rounded together, I still was hoping for a consultative interaction where I could guide and develop local clinicians in their work, rather than being the only physician or clinical officer present as had initially been the case. I knew that I would leave in weeks and that once gone, having been the implementer would have been of short use. I had been told that there was a Sierra Leonan deputy program physician present and others involved in EVD patient care. While that proved not the case, we rounded with nursing staff and discussed case details. He had a ritual to entry as most of us do. Humarr wore a yellow cloth gown set that was placed on him by one of the senior nurses. He walked, arms folded, through the wards making his clinical determinations and issuing medical orders. It was a Herr Doctor Professor approach. He was bright, when he rounded staff was present, and his decisions usually reasonable even when sometimes not what I would have chosen. He had been excited to grow his program to care for EVD patients at the start, I think, as evident by the second ward built and the odd but thoughtful cholera-like beds there. I have worked enough in challenging places to know that hierarchy sometimes is all people have to keep moving when resources are limited. I tried to be careful making suggestions. Humarr would make each one a pronouncement as well.

This was the case when we finished going through doffing our PPE, such as it was. Several staff had been milling about in the shade with laundry. Again, there was no chlorine in the hand washing basin and no one tending the exit area. The hand pump chlorine solution sprayer to decontaminate dirty parts of the PPE before doffing was empty and not easily found. I tried talking and demonstrating to Humarr and again the hygiene staff about the importance of a properly equipped and manned doffing and decontamination station. As on the ward, Humarr probably as a sign of respect reissued my suggestions as pronouncements. There was much direction and subservient response but no movement when the pronouncements continued. Nothing had changed when I rounded alone later that day and the next. Humarr's commanding presence in his local context would not work for me, nor was it effecting changes of behavior.

Humarr's two rounds without me… One day I rounded in the morning in the suspect case ward and met a young girl who had been brought in with her mother. Her mother was ill with EVD and on the confirmed case ward. The girl had a mild fever but otherwise looked well. Her initial test result was negative. She had only just started having a fever, however. At that point we were blessed with a few participatory staff and a nurse who was named French was managing the suspect case ward. He was very conscientious. False negative results on blood PCR testing for Ebola virus can occur commonly up to forty-eight to seventy-two hours after symptom onset. Her first test was negative. I asked that the girl receive empiric therapy for malaria but stay on the ward for testing the next day. She had her own room and bathroom which was quite unusual during that period as we had patients on the floor on other days. The next day, Humarr rounded before me. When French took me around to the rooms in the suspect ward, he told me that the girl had been discharged to the children's ward for malaria therapy as her second test for Ebola virus was negative, but her malaria test was positive. I thought that this was a reasonable decision by Humarr. In retrospect, given the timing of his rounds, he either thought that the previous day's test result was sufficient rather than that an early morning repeat test had been performed, or there simply was confusion about which test result was being discussed. Regardless, the girl was off the wards. I had, the previous night, procured in town some injectable antimalarial medication for her as we were not yet well stocked on the EVD wards. French told me that he had administered one dose the previous night and sent the rest with her to the pediatric ward.

I was very concerned about the possibility of stigma and neglect of this girl who had been just recently discharged from the EVD wards to the pediatric ward. At the time, I thought that there had been two tests for Ebola virus done on her blood and that both had resulted negative. I was very happy that the pediatric ward was staffed and taking patients. Non-EVD services had been patchy at the district hospital while I was there. After rounding on our three wards and doffing PPE, I walked to the pediatric ward. There was a clinical officer in charge. Clinical officers act much like physicians' assistants or perhaps more like independent clinical nurse practitioners in the U.S. I asked to see him, described what I understood about her EVD history and what had been done for her malaria. We discussed how to approach her continued malaria therapy. I left her in what I thought was a better situation than most of my patients.

A couple days later, Mbalu's brother came to see me. He was not a healthcare provider but often was present trying to help at the EVD care center, an extremely unusual practice for the staff other than a few core nurses let alone someone from the community. He had checked in on the girl at the pediatric ward. He told me that she was isolated in a corner of the building and that no one was caring for her.

I went to the ward. She was in an otherwise empty part of the ward. It did not seem that anyone had cared for her since she arrived and the nurse that reluctantly accompanied me to her bedside confirmed that. The girl had not been receiving antimalarial therapy. She was dirty from stool, hot to the touch, and poorly responsive. I suspected that she had both malaria and Ebola virus disease. I went to talk with French at the suspect ward. There was a bed available. He retrieved her in PPE. We started IV fluids and resumed her antimalarial therapy. At first, it seemed that she might respond well to the increased attention. On rounds I typically visited the suspect area first and then went to the confirmed case wards. I am not sure why, maybe avoidance because I knew what I would find, a couple of mornings later I rounded on the confirmed wards first then donned a fresh set of PPE and entered the suspect ward. Hers was the last room I entered. She was awake, uncomfortable making loud grunting noises that did not reach either a cry or a moan. She had blood trickling down the sides of her mouth. She was not moving any limbs. I held her hand and she was able to look at me. Her breathing evened. She stopped making her discomfort sound. I do not know how long I stayed next to her as we looked at each other.

I had rounded for several hours before changing PPE and going to that ward. I knew that I was at my physical limit for the morning. I did not want to leave. I wanted to lie down next to her and let her know that she was not alone. I knew that she was about to die. I did not want to leave her as she died. I did not think that I deserved to leave. I think that had I not left when I did, I would have taken off my PPE and stayed there with her. I walked out of the room without saying anything to French who was outside on a break. The decontamination and doffing area was unmanned which at that moment was just as well. After decontaminating as best as I could and then doffing PPE, I went immediately to the far corner of the hospital compound to an abandoned building project for a new Lassa Fever ward. It usually was vacant. Standing there usually meant that you were alone and able to look either at the burn pit and the hospital wards in one direction, far hills with trees on one side, a field on another and a small community towards the back across a fence. I probably had plenty of reason to cry in Guinea and Sierra Leone before that point, but it was the first time I had done so. It was one of those cries that very young children do that borders on retching and confirms the end of the world. I kicked a rebar from one of the ward's unfinished cement floors, fortunate to not break my foot, then became angry that my foot did not break, that it hurt enough that I could not keep kicking other things and that all of that was distracting me from the girl.

I am not sure what I did for the rest of that day. I thought that perhaps I had reached some kind of normalcy. That was Dan's first day in Kenema. I knew that whatever mask I tried had failed when he asked to speak to me quietly. Mikiko had noticed that something was different and suggested to him that he intercept me. It was venting I needed, well counseled and it did not help me at all feel better, though I resumed my routine afterwards.

The next day the senior technician for handling the mortuary and also for taking blood samples came to me. Though the girl had died the day before, she had not yet been moved to the mortuary. A second test for Ebola virus, as it happens, had never been obtained. Very few people who had died from an undetermined cause were being brought to the hospital then. He was going to take a blood sample. We talked about what approach he was going to use. Apparently, while sometimes he would try to take a sample from the person's heart, he usually simply tried an arm vein, one that typically is used to take routine blood from a patient. Often this would fail as blood clots in small veins quickly. I explained the option of accessing a large, deep vein as an alternative. He looked hesitant but willing and I knew that I needed to demonstrate the procedure to him. I was not looking forward to seeing the girl still, dead. Oddly, coldly, I trained him on the femoral vein collection, drew her blood, coached him on the approach for his future use and we concluded. I was even angrier at myself for having left her after that.

While Humarr may have rounded more frequently than I know, to my knowledge, Humarr's second rounds without me during my time there happened on my last day in Kenema. A U.S. government official conducting an assessment of the response visited the government hospital. Humarr took him into the wards. They were dressed together in PPE, names written clearly on their aprons. This is a good practice generally as it helps patients identify with care providers who are concealed in PPE. In this case, however, it facilitated the photographs being taken of the two of them. I was not with them in the risk area, but when I learned a couple of weeks later that Humarr was infected with EVD, I thought of this event. Maybe in demonstration for the visitor he broke his habit and touched a patient and then himself. He could be very caring. Maybe he simply took care of someone in the community and became infected that way. Maybe as a member of a close-knit healthcare worker community he simply was exposed as a citizen in a setting where the outbreak was happening. It is convenient for me to blame a moment of vanity, instead, as I still am angry at both of us and am not yet feeling charitable, regardless of where fault actually may lie.

The unfinished effort to build a new Lassa Fever ward over the previous few years had its own drama. The program had petitioned to build an innovatively designed ward building that was more functionally organized to replace the hazardous buildings ultimately overrun with EVD patients. The U.S. Embassy took up the project and secured a Navy Facilities contract in order to complete it. An employee of the program in country was the contractor, the same person who managed the program finances. Delays and cost overruns stalled progress and while I was in Kenema it looked like an abandoned, exposed husk. The embassy team was very frustrated by this. I was amazed that it did not become a public embarrassment for everyone involved. Mostly, I was frustrated as the building design well-suited the kind of IPC practice that I was trying to inculcate there. I could not shake the feeling that if it had been in use before the start of the outbreak, processes in general there might have been safer and perhaps there would have been fewer HCW infections amongst the core Lassa Fever Program staff. A close friend of mine was familiar with the Navy Facilities community. I reached out to him from Kenema and he directed me to the cognizant U.S. Navy officers based in Europe. I could get no response from them even when using my U.S. Navy hat. Admittedly, there may be many connectivity and contracting reasons why this would be the case. But, the embassy had no greater luck as it renewed its efforts at the staff level. The presence of this unfinished structure beside the human suffering perpetuated at the EVD care center was obscene.

The laboratory, or rather laboratories, stood in sharp contrast to the wards. The laboratories resided in a similarly older district hospital building but one that had been reasonably maintained. There were offices with doors and window air conditioning units. Two distinct laboratories functioned there—one funded by Tulane and the Lassa Fever Program managed by Augustine Goba and another funded by Metabiota, a contract research organization that specializes in laboratory work for dangerous pathogens, run by Nadia. At the political level, the Tulane-Metabiota programming relationship had been difficult. At the functional level, Lina and Nadia worked quite well together and Augustine often collaborated. Augustine's laboratory had an entire clinical laboratory suite that was not utilized but could provide chemistries and blood count information helpful to patient management. That simply had not been the focus of the laboratory efforts there and they had not yet structured it to handle Ebola virus contaminated specimens. Otherwise, Augustine performed conventional PCR for Ebola and Lassa Fever viruses and at my request malaria rapid testing. Nadia ran a contemporary real time PCR-based assay as well as an antigen-based assay under development by Aileen, Matt and their colleagues in Fort Detrick. There would be conflict around these assays. A PH Canada group had loaded what materials they could on a canoe and made their way from Guinea to Kailahun in order to support diagnostics there. An affable and experienced group, they sought help from Nadia to fill some resulting equipment and reagent gaps. The two laboratory groups disagreed on technical methods. There was discordance between the Kenema PCR assay performance and that of the PH Canada group in one high profile patient investigation and later against a quality control panel. PH Canada like CDC is a key member of the WHO Extremely Dangerous Pathogen Laboratory Network and interested in quality assurance efforts with regards to dangerous pathogen laboratory testing. Whether that single assay tested by the panel was problematic or not is difficult to say. The operational performance of the laboratories, however, seemed predictable and consistent onsite, including when following viral load on admitted patients over the course of their illness. The Kenema laboratories did not rely on any single assay performance. The Tulane and Metabiota laboratories made determinations cooperatively, assessing samples against all three

Ebola virus assays and then adjudicating them collectively, sometimes repeating testing.

I commend the idea of laboratory quality improvement, monitoring and assessment in the field, but think that we too often in high-risk settings ask laboratories to provide either answers to poorly formulated questions or to make assertions that cannot be supported by their tests. We do not let them say a laboratory result is indeterminate, at least that was not the culture in the outbreak in Sierra Leone to do so. Regardless, compared to the remainder of the public health response in Kenema, the laboratories were well resourced. Clearly, they had been well-resourced over time in a program where the obvious focus was laboratory activity. This activity is critical to public health and clinical programming. Though, the best description of the consequences of insufficient clinical investment over the years in that same program is: *catastrophic*.

One of the reasons why laboratories are a common target for investment in these settings is because of control. Once a sample is taken, the sample enters the laboratory space, a closed space in which how the patient and community behave are echoes only. If the right permissions and controls are in place, the samples can be exported to referral centers that can verify and broaden the results, information, yielded from them. Sometimes this happens regardless of the permissions and controls. The Kenema laboratory over the years had built a range of research relationships around sample testing and sharing. Local and international partners benefitted from the sample information and samples themselves from Lassa Fever and other outbreaks assessed through the Kenema program. Research is a tricky topic during the conduct of an outbreak response, however. As I had learned in Guinea and as was reinforced in my brief time in Freetown, the nuances of how research and public health efforts can be synergistic are lost in an environment where trust is not present but fear of exploitation is. Memories of colonial occupation and influences in West Africa are vivid. Some there still believe that U.S. and European modern colonialists created and introduced into Africa the Human Immunodeficiency Virus (HIV) and its deadly clinical syndrome, Acquired Immunodeficiency Syndrome (AIDS). Decades of health risk communication and evidence have not removed this idea. Also, there are globally acknowledged local interests in what happens with sample collection and research. Intellectual property results may generate wealth. While health may be improved by the work, meaningful sharing of products and their resulting wealth may or may not occur. Immediate health concerns may be met but poverty in the at-risk or affected community remains and yet health and public health measures often are a luxury of wealth. The challenge is circular and difficult as advanced technological actors are often important to necessary innovation. Their work is expensive. Yet, international initiatives such as the Pandemic Influenza Preparedness Framework and the Convention on Biological Diversity recognize the importance of benefit sharing. Many people in industry acknowledge this as well as demonstrated by differential pricing of medications for HIV in

Africa in contrast to their higher costs in the U.S. and Europe. The conduct of research as well as the provision of health services around which research occurs both can be complicated.

These complications existed in Kenema. Shortly after my arrival there, one of the core program staff began to be pressured to release public health response information to a foreign research group that had received samples earlier in the outbreak. The person came to me, as I was the senior WHO staff member on the site. The work was not under a protocol for the outbreak, specifically, and so it had not been vetted for human protection concerns in that context. Also, I did not have a Ministry of Health point of contact with whom I could coordinate release of the information. The research group had written permission for their work leading up to this request, but it was not clear that it had been obtained by or structured in the usual ways for research under the rules from the Government of Sierra Leone. I sought support from the larger WHO response team. The research may have been perfectly valid and the information apt to it, but I believed that it was for a Ministry of Health official to make that determination, to request that information from the response team and deliver it to the researchers. Ideally, the MoH would have the opportunity to assess carefully all requests from groups seeking samples and other Sierra Leone information for export. They should be able to balance their varied interests and make it work for them and the researchers. This was the way that the response team and MoH in Guinea managed to move past their consequential shut down in the spring. I did not want to be complicit in causing the same such interruption of activities in Sierra Leone.

Unfortunately, though perhaps validating my concerns by inaction, no one with the appropriate authority accepted responsibility in the conversation. The drama of the event increased as local and international people involved in the Lassa Fever program sought to fire this whistleblower. The person had acted completely appropriately, had done so in a way that left open the possibility of everyone's needs being met and was critical to the public health response. Fortunately, the Sierra Leone government officials understood this. My energy shifted from trying to find a way to accommodate the researchers to interrupting the attempt at retribution on the whistleblower. Later I saw the most contentious of the data reflected plainly in a very high-profile publication that included the involved parties. In the end, the researchers must simply have taken advantage of our poor security at the care center or managed to get the data from someone else more accommodating though no more authorized. At first, I considered various regulatory means to deal with the offenders in their own country. In the end, though, the whistleblower was still employed and had sublimated most of the events; their paper, though with some technical issues, was not more egregious in its identifiable detail of affected communities (one of my principal concerns related to the lack of review that had occurred in an acute event where tribes and villages act out against each other) than soon to follow WHO papers by some of my colleagues; maybe in the long view that kind of detail is important; the research group's behavior was obnoxious but not unheard of for actors in field research on dangerous pathogens and in other international health research; even if all that occurred to me as possible about the way the work came together was true, it was more opportunistic than illegal; the event was emblematic of the oddness of the relationships and work that developed in Kenema over years. So, I merely recused myself from related publications.

We were very disconnected from the larger WHO response team operating out of northern Kailahun. In addition to not receiving support on the research issues from Freetown or the northern Kailahun team, we also had very little understanding of their broader challenges or performance. When I would visit Daru to support Ibrahim, Alpha, and their team, I would hear a little bit about activities north. We were too overwhelmed in Kenema to lose me, Chris, or Mikiko to make an overnight trip in order to be able to interact with them and return. Knowing the disparate caseloads at the time, we wondered at the preponderance of WHO resources that they had. They also had taken with them several staff from the Lassa Fever program prior to my arrival. That said, under optimal circumstances, they probably were understaffed for the work as they saw it and may have done better than us by leveraging more resources for less acute need to longer effect. That is my sublimation.

Initially, I assumed that the MSF-led EVD care center in Kailahun was providing the same kind of reach back support and mentorship for the transitional care center in Koindu, near the border with Guinea, that Tom and then I tried to provide to the one in Daru. I had no knowledge of the composition of the MSF clinical team in Kailahun. I had tried repeatedly to reach their coordinator by mobile telephone without success. There were several topics I wanted to discuss with that person, ranging from mutual support to Daru, Koindu and medevac patterns. This made their brief appearance and rapid departure early on when I was in the suspect case ward all the more frustrating. Eventually I decided that I should call Koindu simply to say hello. Even if Koindu was well supported by the other EVD care center, samples still found their way to us for testing somehow, even with the PH Canada laboratory by then running in Kailahun, and I could assist in getting results or just general technical questions.

Mobile telephone service was patchy while I was in Kenema. Reaching Ibrahim in Daru or colleagues in Freetown was a constant challenge. Remarkably, I reached the Koindu clinical officer on the first try and the first ring. The clinical officer told me that Koindu, fortunately, had received an initial MSF water-sanitation consultation and assistance in getting structured. The clinical officer said that he was not interacting with the MSF clinical team, however. We spoke briefly about how he was and the work of the unit. My sense was that like Daru, Koindu was an important evaluation and sample collection site, with less staff but also less patient burden than in Daru. He was busy, but at the time of the call he said that the workload was in a steady stream and that the ambulances taking patients to the MSF site ran reliably. He called me the next night to talk more. He had been feeling ill for several days. He was tired and it felt a bit like malaria when last he had it. We discussed his care, including taking fluid and presumptive treatment for malaria, as well as the importance that he not place himself at risk by trying to continue work in PPE while feeling ill. Slowly we got to the point in the conversation where I felt like he would be ready to discuss the possibility that he had EVD. He was ahead of me. He had sent a sample of his own blood for testing in Kailahun a few days before. I told him that I would check for the result and that he should consider finding a ride to the MSF site. He said that one would be available the next day.

When we hung up the phone, I went to the laboratory to speak with Nadia. She spent several minutes with me scouring the sample records. For some reason, a sample from the Koindu clinical officer had just come to Kenema. I am not sure if it was sent as part of quality assurance or diverted because of some capacity issue in Kailahun. Regardless, she had it and it was running. Quickly, she was able to let me know that the sample tested positive for Ebola virus. I called and informed him. We talked for a while about how to approach his own care. He also promised to take the morning ambulance to the MSF site. For hours afterwards I tried to reach either the MSF or WHO staff in Kailahun so that they could ensure that the clinical officer made the trip safely and received care. In the end, an epidemiologist on the

WHO team there received the message. I heard later that the Koindu clinical officer and the MSF team were successful in his care. He eventually returned to Koindu and resumed his work with suspect EVD patients.

While Dan was in Freetown advising the larger response team he managed to do something both Tom and I had tried but not managed to do, namely convince the MoH that it was in its best interest to pull healthcare staff from around the country and have it rotate through Kenema. The convincing argument was the scale of the outbreak. The outbreak had grown to the point where more robust planning in Freetown was required, not just for a sentinel case or two but the possibility of several cases from urban transmission had occurred in Conakry. The MoH reticence to do this initially was frustrating but understandable. Sierra Leone has very few healthcare workers. Durable health threats are realized in every community, and diversion of staff to the outbreak meant enlarging already present gaps elsewhere. Nonetheless, planning was underway for an EVD care center at Lakka outside Freetown at the site of a tuberculosis hospital. It had to be staffed. The idea was to bring prospective staff through Kenema for familiarization and training enroute Lakka and other sentinel isolation sites around the country.

As happy as I was that Dan was successful in this, there were challenges. First, while Kenema remained the principal patient care site to which suspect and confirmed patients were sent from across the country save the northern Kailahun catchment, Kenema's capacity had collapsed. Key members of the original Lassa Fever Program clinical staff had started becoming ill with Ebola. Patients outnumbered beds. Staff that were available were only variably paid and sometimes threatened enough during their commute that they could not present for work. Support staff continued not to be present or when present engaged and so remotely appropriate water, sanitation and hygiene were constant challenges. When Dan arrived, in addition to the challenge I presented that day after we lost that girl, he was faced with a reality in Kenema quite different than the program in its heyday that he helped to develop years ago.

Dan's arrival in Kenema gave Chris, Mikiko, and me several opportunities. He was able to say the things we had been saying anew; say things we had not; and also rely on and mediate from relationships he had developed in Kenema over years. In short, he was equipped to be efficient and effective getting both our local colleagues and partners in the field to take measures we had been requesting. When a small resurgence in staff coverage occurred, he was able to get them together with their non-EVD care center leadership for training and to review safe practice procedures in ways that I had not been able to do.

Visits to Kenema were rare. Most people did not wish to be close to the EVD care center. Two instances contrasted sharply. The first was from a representative from the larger U.N. country team. He came to the district medical officer but not to the care site. As in my first meeting in Freetown, he was interested in identifying a quick purchase that could be made, seen to be delivered into east Sierra Leone branded with U.S. symbols as a single contribution. I was desperately in need of logistics support to include an improvement in the flow of MoH resources to the district from Freetown and in particular, healthcare worker salaries, insurance and risk pay so that we could have enough people on the ward to make the environment safer and more effective. We did not arrive at a useful common ground. The second visit was far more interesting. Keiji came to Sierra Leone from Geneva. He was traveling to each of the affected countries. This was shortly before WHO Headquarters started interacting more directly with the outbreak leading to a Public Health Emergency of International Concern (PHEIC) determination. I knew Keiji well from working in his office in Geneva, and seeing him helped me feel more connected to life before Kenema. The northern Kailahun team came south for the meeting. Keiji was patient and genuinely interested in the work. Chris, Mikiko, and Lina who were so crucial to the larger public health response in Kenema and southern Kailahun finally had a hearing for the many challenges of operating independently with little on-site support or reach back to Freetown. Perhaps most importantly, Keiji was able to appreciate the growing scale and diversity of the outbreak.

Dan and I were grateful when Dr. Alie Wurie from the MoH delivered several transplanted staff intended for the pending facility at Lakka. Dan led classroom sessions with them along with a WHO deployed

IPC specialist, and then Dan and I took them in teams to familiarize and embed them in ward work. Two more WHO deployed clinical consultants arrived. Rob had managed to cobble together rotations for clinical coverage for Kenema for the rest of the summer. Dr. Tim O'Dempsey from the Liverpool School of Tropical Medicine and Dr. Takayu Adachi from Toshima Hospital in Tokyo were obviously well trained and experienced clinicians. By the time Tim and Takuya arrived, they were to experience a very different start than me and then Dan. Staff was present and more organizational procedures were being observed. Ultimately, they would experience some of the same kinds of fluctuations and capacity challenges that we did. Tim later returned to Sierra Leone in order to provide important leadership to the clinical response in Freetown through Save the Children and other health groups.

As my arrangements to leave Sierra Leone were getting sorted, I suggested to Geneva that they move me directly from Kenema to Lofa, Liberia. Samaritan's Purse, a faith-based NGO that works in West Africa among other places, and its partners had been the first non-MSF care provisioning entities to engage in the outbreak. We still had not managed to get anyone to assess and assist the operation there. The degree of the outbreak in Liberia still was poorly characterized. Between Geneva and the newly forming operations node for the U.N. Mission for Ebola Emergency Response (UNMEER) in Accra, no one could arrange entrée into Liberia for me, so my arrangements remained through Freetown to Geneva. That was my second strike in trying to get to Liberia.

On my last day in Kenema, Alex came to see me just outside the care center. He looked tired and was in street clothes. He told me that he felt tired and ill, similar to when he had had malaria. We talked for a while, both aware of what this might mean. He insisted on going home but went first to have blood drawn for both Ebola virus and malaria testing. I gave him money to buy anti-malaria medication from the local pharmacy. He was not having diarrhea, but we discussed how to manage his fluid status initially until he came to the care center should it develop. We verified that we had each other's correct mobile telephone numbers, and I said goodbye to him. I warned Dan and Lina about the conversation.

Departing the next morning was an odd experience. Chris, Mikiko, and I had become very close with late night data work fueled by alcohol into the small hours. I also had come to know Dan well quite quickly. Tim and Takuya seemed so new to the field despite all of their other experiences. Five hours later I was in Freetown. I might as well have been an ocean away.

Returning to Freetown meant a swirl of response team meetings. Dr. Joseph Fair, a former colleague of Dan's, was assisting with Emergency Operations Center (EOC) activities at the WHO country office. They were well run but like high-level meetings in any country, it was hard to see the connections to activity on the ground. While hoping for travel arrangements to Liberia but waiting for a flight back to Geneva, I started roving to make preparatory site visits at major medical centers in and near Freetown. I worked with Dr. Marta Llado at Connaught Hospital demonstrating the femoral vein sampling technique on a deceased suspect case and also running through general procedures. It seemed a very good but small shop. There was a private Indian hospital that had developed a decent two-bed capacity for sentinel cases. They still were reeling as an MSF provider with malaria had recently been sent there for care pending return to Europe. Apparently, International SOS, the contracted medevac service, had declined to collect the patient once they suspected EVD. Fortunately, the provider did not have EVD and apparently had fared well, returning to work. There was a large hospital called Friendship Hospital in the city's outskirts. It was a gift of the Chinese government and staffed with a mix of Chinese and Sierra Leone healthcare workers. While they reported a high number of cases for usual referral hospital care, the facility was almost empty like most I had seen during this period. They had set aside a couple of rooms for potential isolation of two to three EVD suspected cases in one of the buildings. However, they had not taken an opportunity yet to develop and walk through procedures. The staff was very welcoming, and I understand ultimately provided some EVD care. In particular, I was interested in Lakka, the site intended for the staff in training at Kenema. When I went, it was incomplete and with no staff, equipment, or supplies. While next to a national reference laboratory for influenza and HIV testing, that laboratory had not been enlisted for participation in the response. The site had not advanced since Dan had provided technical advice during his time in Freetown. The MSF country director helpfully provided some water and sanitation recommendations. He later shared those recommendations with me. I renewed his and Dan's recommendations as well as additional ones. I suggested that just as all affected areas should be seeking foreign medical team support to work in concert with national staff, that this would be a good site for a deployable laboratory, perhaps South Africa. Ultimately, both of these things happened.

In the midst of this, one EOC meeting stands out in my mind. Suspect cases were beginning to occur more frequently in western areas of Sierra Leone. A relatively affluent foreign businessman with long-term interests in Sierra Leone apparently had become infected, managed to evade the travel restrictions on departing Kenema, and arrived at a small private hospital in Freetown. That hospital concealed him from public health authorities. He had died and a public health investigation was underway to attempt to identify potential contacts at risk for infection close to the city. The conversation grew to the preparedness status of Freetown, which I had just assessed, and the in-place sample and patient transport strategy to Kenema. The Minister of Health was present. I do not find meetings helpful as a general rule and am loathe to speak in them, probably a sign of an underlying immaturity on my part. However, the Ministry and their partners statements about the convenience of Kenema concerned me, particularly in the context of my persistent reporting to the contrary about Kenema's appropriateness while there and since return to Freetown. I told the Minister bluntly that Kenema is completely unsustainable. Kenema should be either closed or control transferred to an appropriately resourced foreign medical team experienced in the care of patients in emergencies with substantial logistical, water and sanitation support. The room became quiet for a couple moments, there was some nodding, and then, ultimately after my departure, my statement was ignored. The national response strategy still relied on national medevac and sample referral to a collapsed or, in variably improved periods collapsing, Kenema EVD care center.

While in Freetown I had several calls from eastern Sierra Leone. Humarr called me a few times to talk about the research issues. They were, I think, cordial and constructive conversations. Chris, Mikiko, Dan, and I spoke to update each other. Then I received a call from Lina. Alex was infected with Ebola virus and becoming progressively ill. Calls quickly followed from Chris and Mikiko. Alex and I spoke. Initially, his spirits were good. Mbalu, however, followed him into the isolation ward as a patient. I called Alex frequently. He became less and less interactive on the telephone. Alex asked me when I was going to be coming back to Kenema. I desperately wanted to find a driver and return. Not doing so was the second hardest thing I have ever done, after walking away from that girl on the suspect case ward. I cannot believe still that I did not go to Kenema and care for Alex. I kept thinking that I cannot, Dan and Tim and Takuya are there. They are good physicians. The last thing that they need or that the patients need is for me to sweep through pretending to be more useful than the greater talent that they had pooled there. They needed space to do what they do. I also was not sure that I was safe in that environment without a break. All feedback I received later says that they did well—they were conscientious, caring clinicians. Even though I appreciate that it is not rational to do so, I still blame myself.

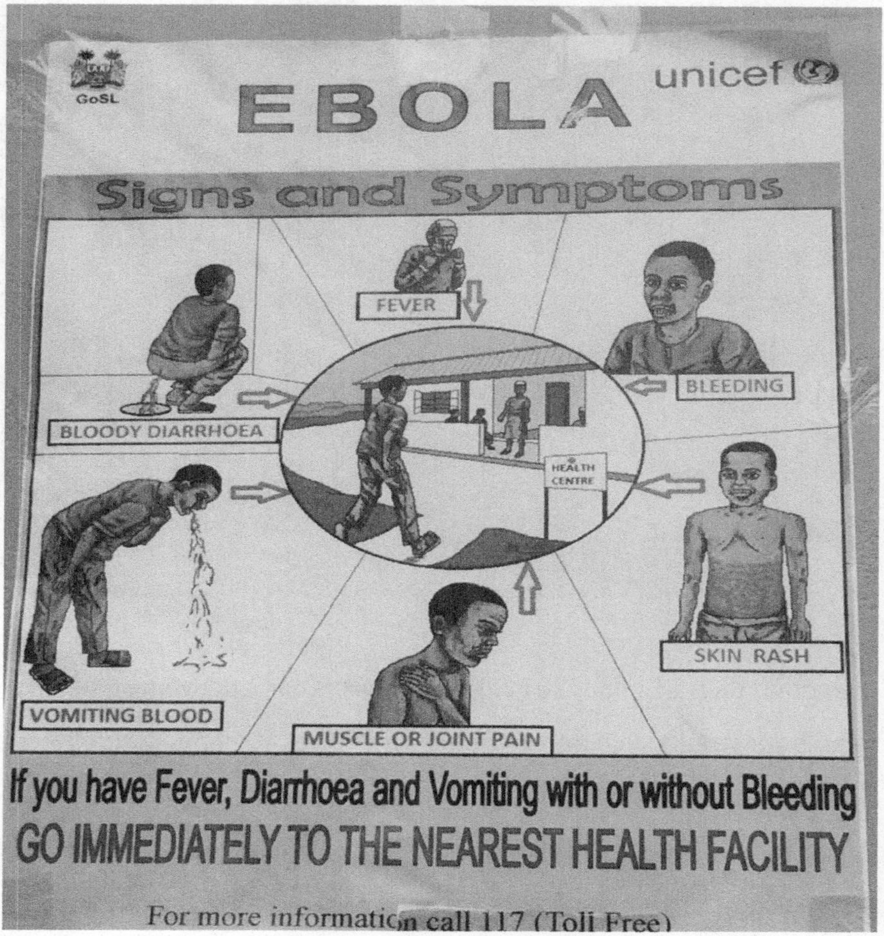

Photo courtesy of Dr. Mikiko Senga. Kenema, Sierra Leone, 2014.

Blunt messaging abounded.

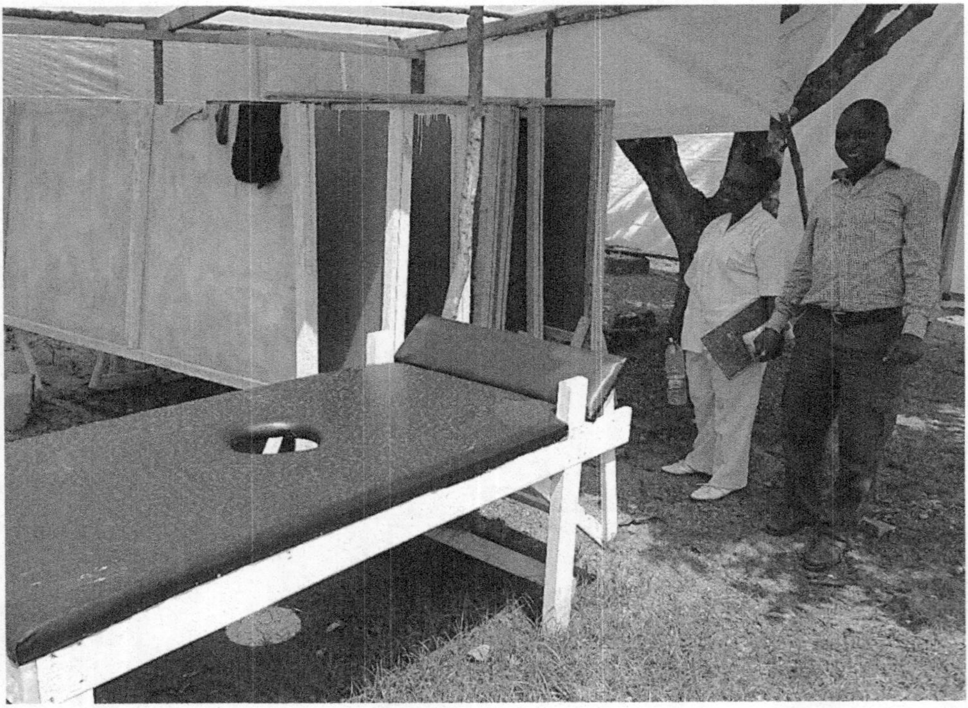

Kenema, Sierra Leone, 2014. Dr. Humarr Khan and Matron Mbalu, who both would succumb to Ebola virus disease, show their cholera-like bed to allow stool collection while a patient is supine. Unfortunately, neither sufficient staff or buckets would be available to make use of this hygiene feature.

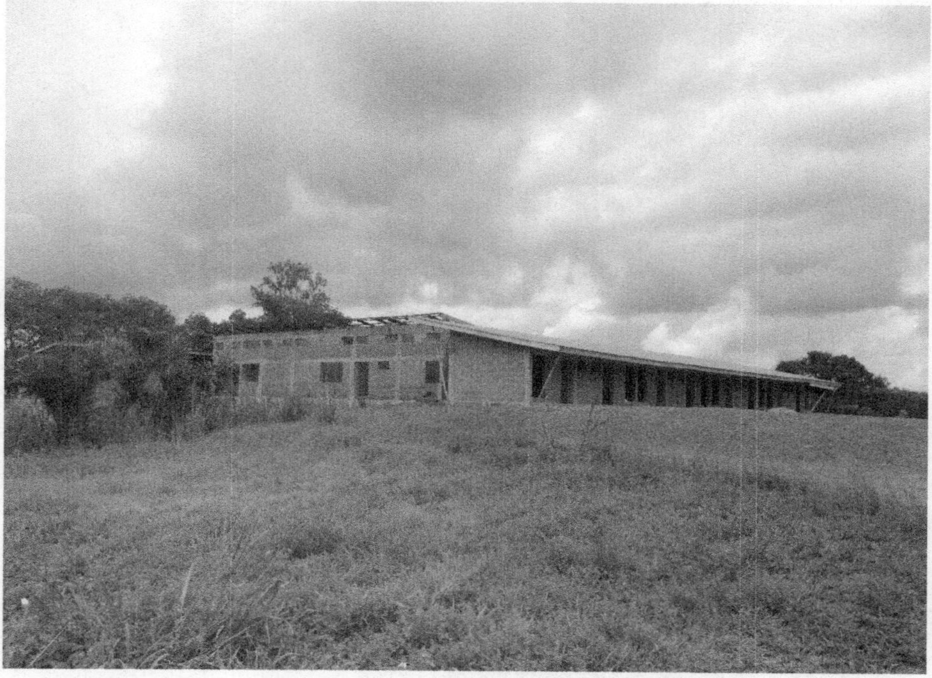

Photo courtesy of Dr. Mikiko Senga, Kenema, Sierra Leone, 2014. The would-be Lassa Fever ward that never was, would have assisted greatly in the EVD outbreak.

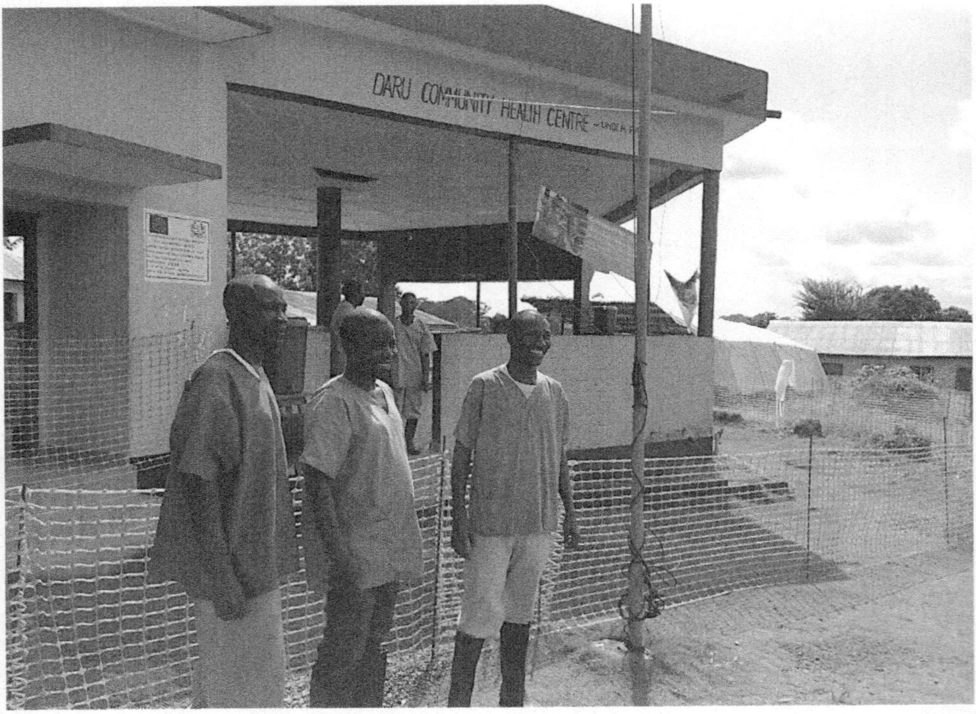

Photo courtesy of Dr. Mikiko Senga, Kenema, Sierra Leone, 2014. The incredibly hard-working Ibrahim and Alpha at the Daru transition center, helping southern Kailahun District with triage and community outreach in the outbreak.

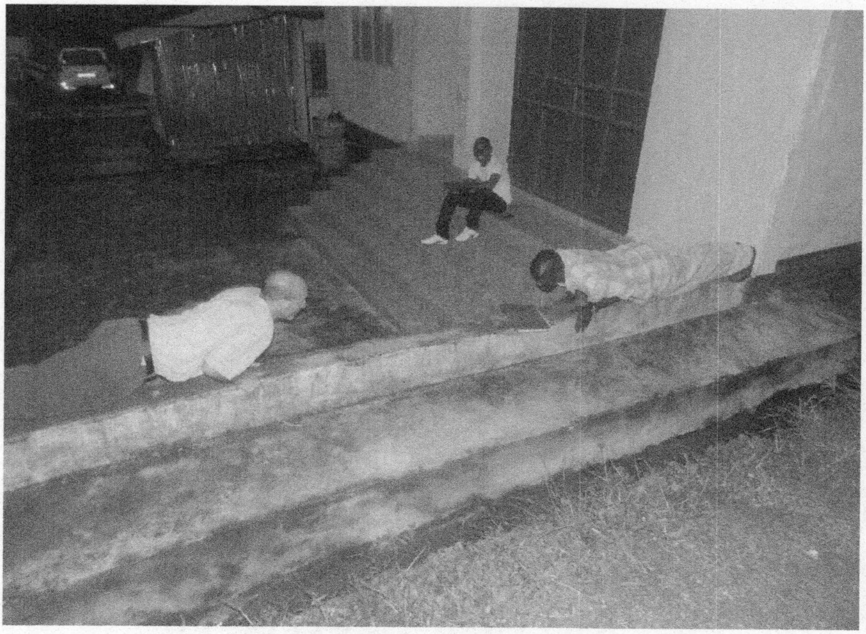

Photo courtesy of Dr. Jimmy Kapetshi, Sierra Leone, 2014. Jimmy deployed in support of the diagnostic laboratory on-site in Kenema. While waiting for our ride late at night, he saw me teaching some Sierra Leone colleagues a game from the Naval Academy. Every time the story teller says “down,” all drop, when “up,” all push up. The stories could last a while.

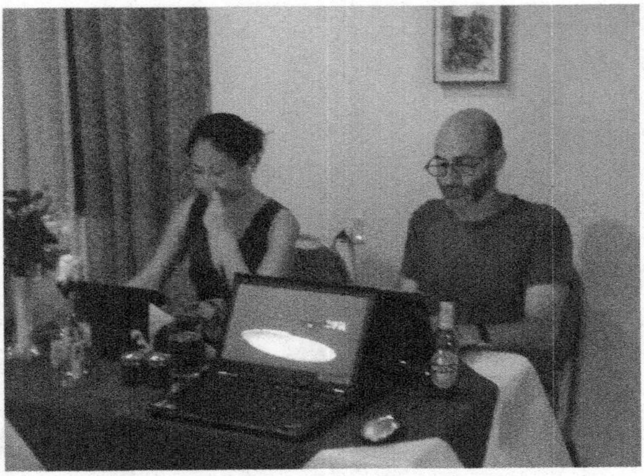

Photo courtesy of Mr. Chris Lane, Sierra Leone, 2014. Midnight meant rare connectivity for Mikiko, Chris, and I.

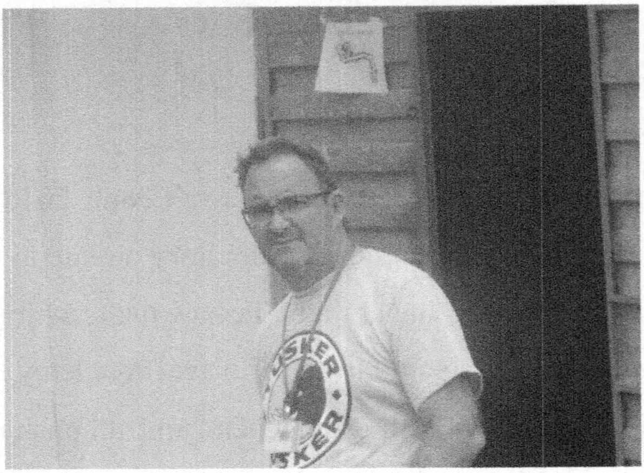

Photo courtesy of Mr. Chris Lane, Sierra Leone, 2014. Super effective and always moving, Kenyan Chris proudly displays his home country's well known lager.

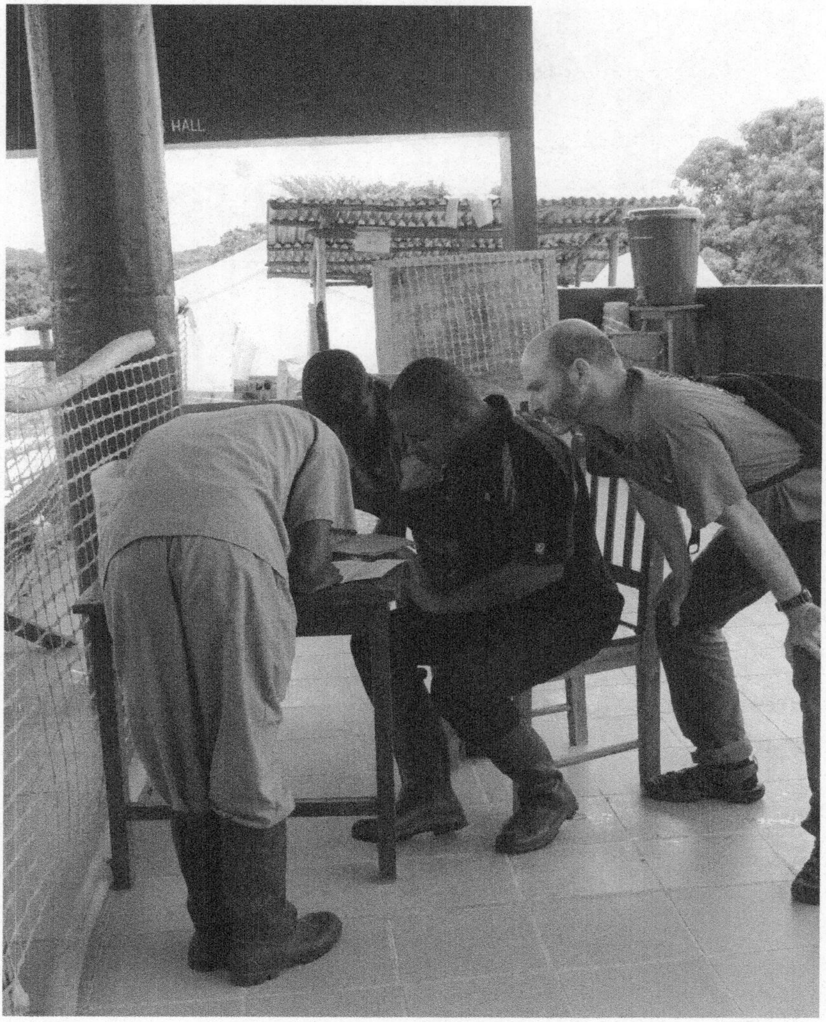

Photo courtesy of Mr. Chris Lane, Sierra Leone, 2014. In Daru, Ibrahim and I sort their patient log with his team.

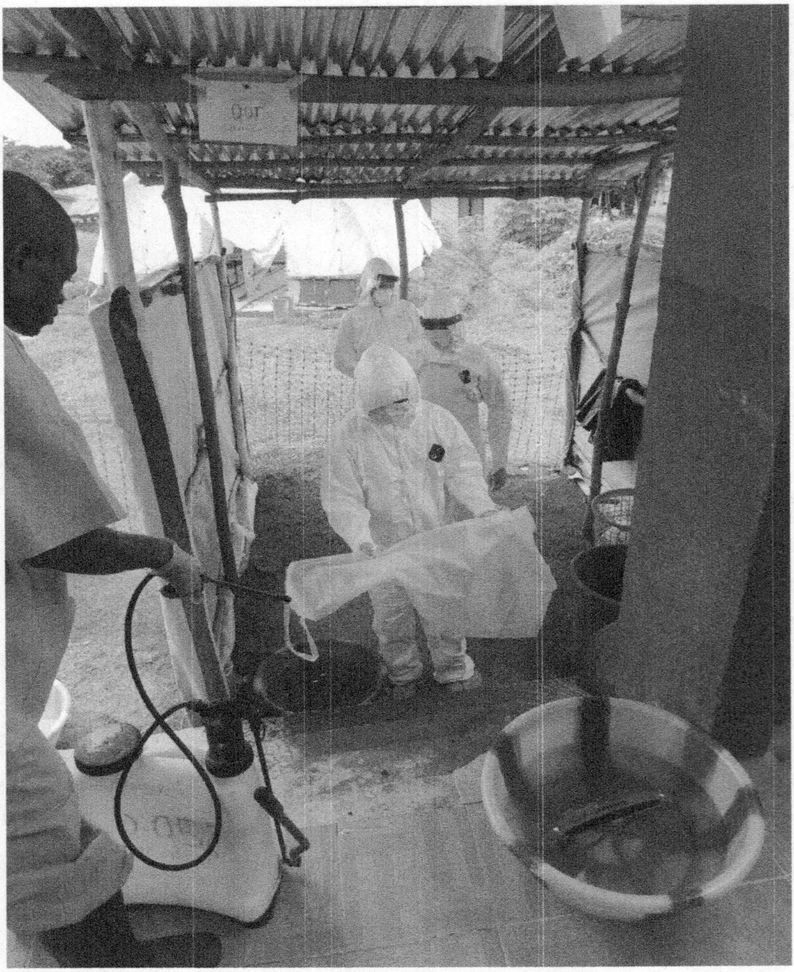

Photo courtesy of Mr. Chris Lane, Sierra Leone, 2014. I am last in the queue to doff PPE when I hear a noise from a tent behind me that I thought was empty. I gave Chris some tense moments as I went back halfway through doffing into the high-risk area to try and get a small child there to drink ORS.

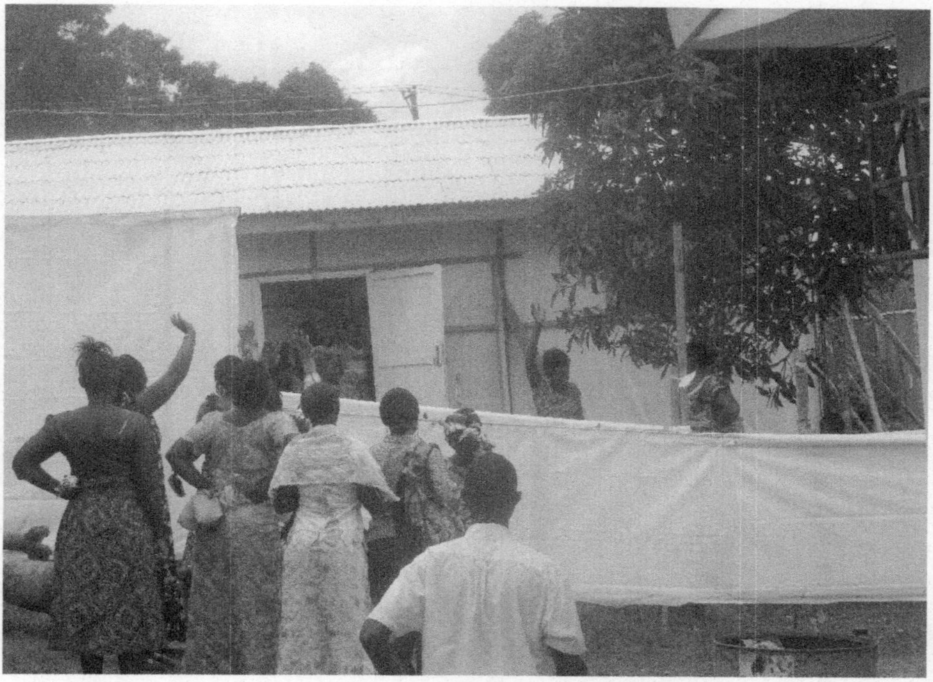

Photo courtesy of Mr. Chris Lane, Sierra Leone, 2014. In Kenema, occasionally there was a nice moment with a recovering patient and community visit.

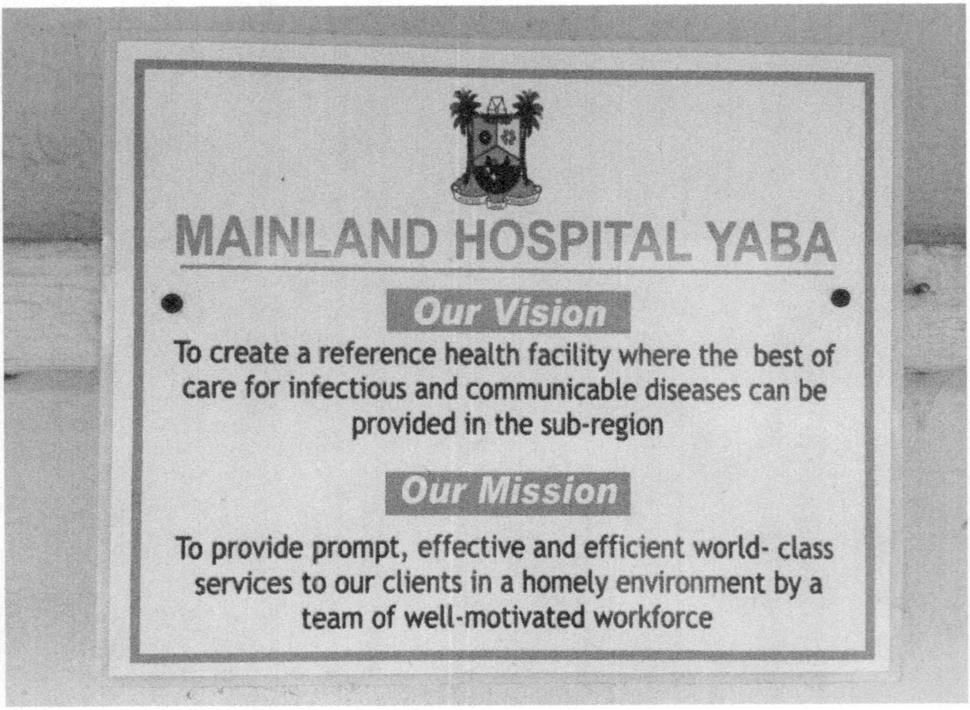

Lagos, Nigeria, 2014. The mission of Mainland Hospital Yaba where essentially all triage and care in Lagos would occur for Ebola virus disease (EVD) during the outbreak was both aspirational and ironic.

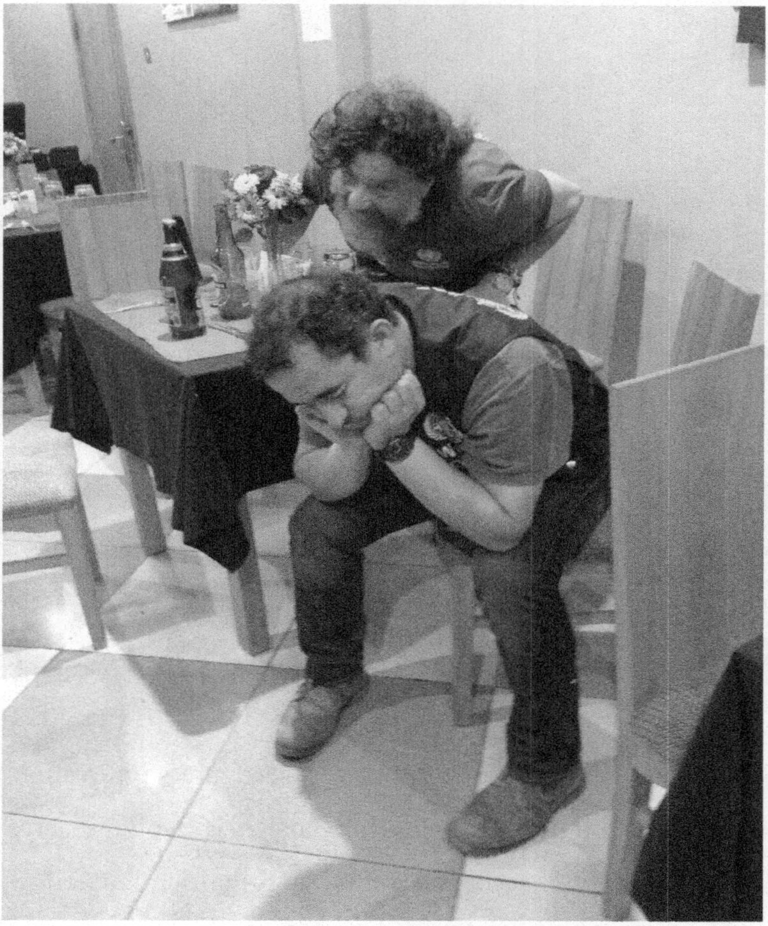

Lagos, Nigeria, 2014. Even the formidable logistician Kamal Ait-Ikhlef eventually suffered the consequences of routinely dining at midnight. Posing unbeknownst to Kamal is WHO colleague Dr. Maurizio Barbeschi.

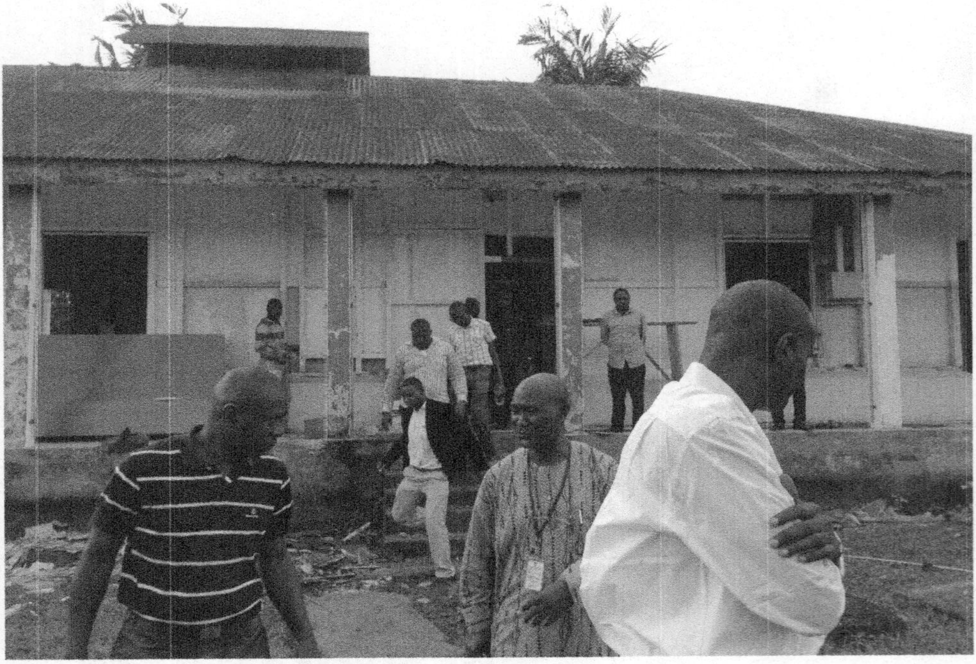

Lagos, Nigeria, 2014. Work began on this structure's renovation for use as an isolation ward shortly after my arrival. It would receive many resources but not see a patient. In the foreground in yellow and blue is the Mainland Clinic director, Dr. Gbadamosi.

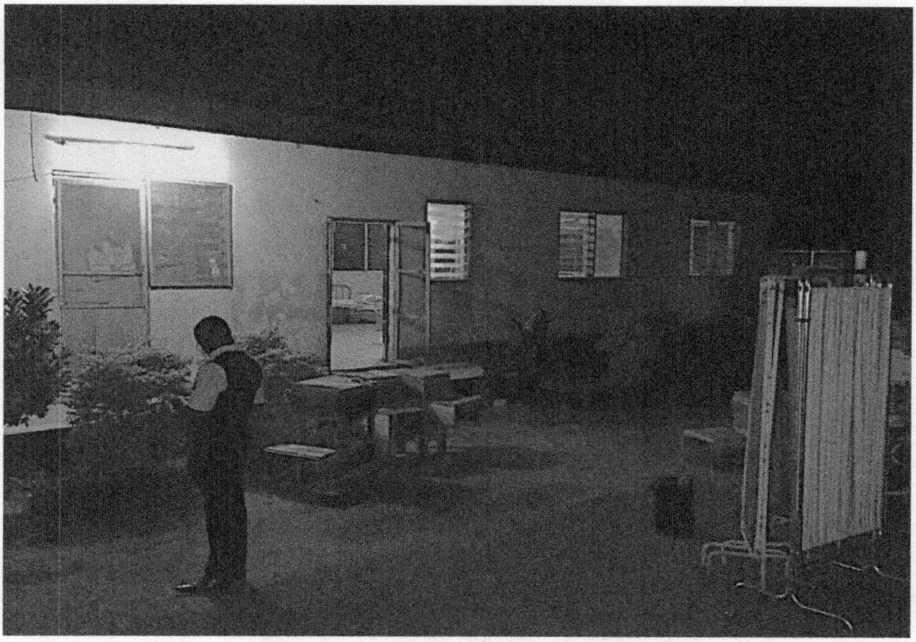

Lagos, Nigeria, 2014. Before the newer tuberculosis ward was adopted for the care of EVD patients shortly before I departed, patient care was conducted in this long-abandoned building. Dr. Emmanuel Musa (WHO) stands in front just after we all set to work clearing and cleaning it for the patient waiting in the ambulance. Its layout forced very unorthodox workflows.

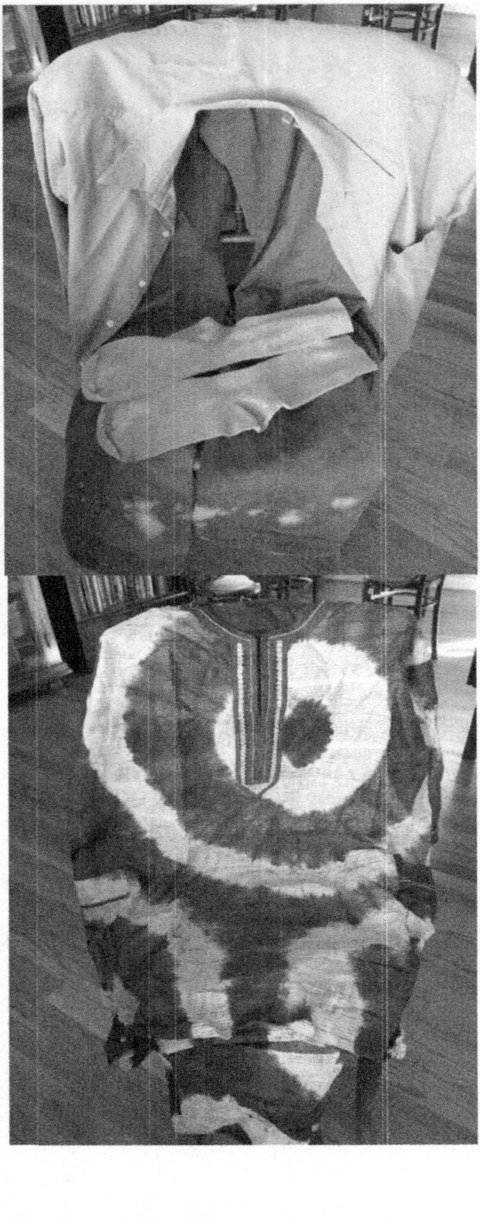

Bleach had taken a toll on my wardrobe while in Nigeria. The Governor's medical lead kindly provided me some local dress.

Nigeria

"The naked traveller,

Stretching, against the iron dawn, the bowstrings of his eyes,

Starves on the mad sierra."

-Thomas Merton in "Ash Wednesday", *New Selected Poems of Thomas Merton*

“Speaking from Havana, WHO Director-General Margaret Chan called the outbreak the world’s worst ever by number of cases, saying, ‘The situation is serious but not out of control yet.’” “Ebola death toll in Africa jumps to 603”, *The Huffington Post*, July 15, 2014

“Ebola reaches Nigeria with death of Liberian” Al Jazzera, July 25, 2014

“U.S. doctor working in Liberia contracts Ebola” *The Telegraph*, July 27, 2014

“It was the unanimous view of the Committee that the conditions for a Public Health Emergency of International Concern (PHEIC) have been met.” *WHO Disease Outbreak News*, August 8, 2014

Returning to Geneva from Sierra Leone was a bit different than after Conakry. I had a larger sense of risk from the environment in Kenema. Our house had a basement bedroom and bathroom. I was more meticulous about only using that bathroom and sleeping downstairs until I had been away from Kenema for two weeks. My exposures in Freetown were minimal and the environment more controlled. A few days after I returned there was a clinical management working meeting at WHO. Dan had returned to Geneva by then. Rob and Shevin were there, as were Christophe and Francois, Dan's wife and colleague, Frederique, some friends and colleagues from MSF Suisse and other stakeholders. It was a small meeting. It seemed to focus on rehashing existing educational programming on treating adults with sepsis, severe illness from an infection. That was not necessarily bad, and it remains important work. I was frustrated, though. I could not see the clinical response developing that I thought was needed, a larger strategy applied for more robust workforce, true monitoring, assessment and intervention, coordinated team activity. That is not to say that my colleagues were not doing that, it simply was not visible to me. I was angry and reacted strongly with an old prejudice of mine against people talking about training in the developing world as though it is a great gift even when not matched with human and other resources to allow it be practiced safely and effectively, or when uncoupled from the longer term relationships that allow mentorship and progress. Training sessions detached from any real strategic programming to change medium- and long-term health outcomes are the low hanging fruit grabbed by most of us from the tree of global health opportunity. I was too angry to couch any of these concerns constructively. Instead, I railed unhelpfully to the group a bit, grunted, beat the ground with a club, and managed to get disinvited from most subsequent processes.

A couple of months later, when I was asked to step in to help coordination a bit, Dan sent me an e-mail that said, "You really are very good at what you do, you just need to figure out how to not make people so mad when you do it." The latter was a fair criticism that I probably should have discerned and heeded many years ago. Even when angry, though, usually my more abrupt messages are because I assume that most people around me have already arrived at the same observations I have in my head, even if they weigh them in importance differently. This happened that same week in the Strategic Health Operations Center (SHOC). My Alert and Response colleagues asked me to provide a debriefing on my time in Sierra Leone. I had not been asked to do this after returning from Conakry. As I felt that clinical care and public health coordination were one of the outstanding gaps in the response, I said yes. In referring to the challenges in better coordination, I mentioned the various forms of drama that had occurred around laboratories. The unsaid agreement that laboratory quality assurance is important but with challenges of context in my head behind my quip, "and the laboratory drama was crap," was lost. I immediately was set upon about the fundamental importance of laboratories and my clear lack of understanding of how testing is used. Fortunately, and against my usual practice, I managed to exert just enough frontal inhibition to not respond, not to point out that their reaction was a perfect example of the lopsided, disconnected view preparedness and response teams, research groups, aid and development agencies, and many others have of the role of laboratories. They then offered, "Well, some say that when MSF runs an EVD care center, staff live, and when WHO does it, they die." I think that I responded successfully, or at least deliberately, parsing the difference between WHO dropping in to help local staff in their efforts while awaiting and advocating for the arrival of resources and foreign medical teams to the deliberate effort of a properly resourced clinical provisioning entity like MSF. I also suspect that I am the only one in the SHOC for that session that remembers, perseverates on that conversation, and realizes how close we came to bloodshed.

At home, we planned for an overdue vacation. My wife's grandmother had emigrated as a girl from Alsace. While we were in touch with cousins who lived in other parts of France, we had not yet been to Alsace. We planned a few days in Strasbourg, a day's drive from Geneva, and were thinking about extending it to a few days ambling about the countryside. We had managed to do a few weekend trips but had not yet been able to really take advantage of our time in central Europe. I finally was reaching fourteen days post-Kenema. When I had returned from Guinea, I was somewhat cavalier about the potential infection risk for Ebola that I might pose to others. My experience in Sierra Leone, however, was far less resourced and constrained. While I did not feel ill, I slept in our basement guestroom and always used that bathroom. I was cautious about physical contact. Also, I had taken an antimalarial drug to prevent contracting malaria in both Guinea and Sierra Leone. This is important when traveling to malaria-infected mosquito-laden areas. This also is important when deploying into an Ebola outbreak where malaria is present. Having a fever from malaria forces an evaluation for EVD that includes isolation. In Guinea, I had taken a drug called Malarone and tolerated it well. In Sierra Leone, however, I experienced a known and problematic side effect, oral ulcers. They became so bad while in Sierre Leone that I stopped eating, resolving quickly when I stopped my Malarone. I had mefloquine with me, another antimalarial drug. However, mefloquine can cause dream disturbance and mood changes, so I did not think that it was compatible with my state of mind there. I had become a non-adherent patient and was a little concerned that I might falsely become a suspect EVD patient. Most cases of EVD result in symptoms within ten days of exposure, so I was relieved to be reaching two weeks.

On the road to Strasbourg on Friday, July 25, we got a call. WHO was about to post a formal notification by the Nigeria National Focal Point that there was a probable EVD patient in Lagos. Federal and state officials in Nigeria were organizing an interagency response team. WHO was looking for people who could deploy over the weekend to provide support. Lagos is a major metropolitan area with significant health resources in contrast to the currently affected areas of West Africa. The purpose of the mission was to provide technical advice as the Nigerians began contact tracing and monitoring and also to explore other areas of preparedness. They wanted a clinician on the team. I agreed to leave on Monday. The patient in question already had died. He had received care in what was reported to be a well-staffed private hospital with IPC procedures in place and PPE supplies. Even in the middle of a PHEIC, WHO, just like most large government bureaucracies, has trouble putting together international travel orders and arrangements on weekends. Actually, I had been lobbying and still felt that it was a higher priority for me to get to Liberia. I had failed twice in getting there. We had not fielded clinical consultants to Samaritan's Purse yet. I had just returned home from Sierra Leone and had not spent any real time with my wife, Shelly, and the girls until we got into the car that morning. We briefly enjoyed Strasbourg.

Shelly remained patient with my Ebola-related deployments, though increasingly less enamored with my doing them. She was more-or-less ambivalent about my going to Sierra Leone. Now, however, she was unhappy but resigned. Later, she revealed to me that she was quite concerned. In over twenty years of service in the U.S. Navy, my time in Sierra Leone and Nigeria was the first time that she was worried about my safety in more than an abstract fashion. It was not because of Ebola virus. Shelly had experienced several different kinds of deployments. Early in our marriage in 1993, as a sea-going junior officer and long before I would become a physician, I was a member of the Maritime Interdiction Force, a shipboard collateral duty. As part of NATO Operation Sharp Guard, we boarded ships in the Adriatic Sea to ensure adherence to U.N. Security Council resolutions against arms importation into Yugoslavia. Shelly did not know this until while I was deployed, when another Navy wife said that she had heard that I was "M.I.A." Shelly thought that those sorts of notifications came from uniformed personnel who arrive at the door via a black sedan. She was more surprised when the woman said that she had a video. With trepidation, she watched it. There on the screen before her, I emerged with my weapon over the railing of a merchant ship at sea. Her friend had mistook "M.I.F." for "M.I.A," missing in action. The video had been taken by a senior chief petty officer also on the team. Shelly was experienced with my doing foolish and dangerous things when deployed. The chaotic, unsupported nature of my time in Sierra Leone is what worried her, and foreshadowed my experience in Nigeria. My youngest daughter, then five years old, had a simpler view. "Will you be taking care of children?" "Possibly." "Well, go, but then come back."

Still in the background, brewing drama about my assignment to WHO lurked. The Navy had not yet acknowledged the extension request from WHO. People in Washington remained distracted on the subject. Questions inside Navy Medicine and throughout the U.S. Government were starting to circulate about which agencies might participate in a larger, more committed U.S. response. And, despite my reports, no one really understood what I had been doing in the field.

On Monday, July 28, a little more than a week after I had left Sierra Leone, I was in Lagos.

I was contacted by Alastair MacKenzie in late September, 2015. He played my character in a Nigerian production called *93 Days* done in cooperation with some independent studios in the U.S. and U.K. The movie focuses on physicians who managed the first known Ebola patient in Lagos, and later became ill from the disease. Alastair sent me an e-mail at the beginning of filming. He had just arrived in Lagos. His e-mail was the first notice I had received of the movie. He suffered what probably was a horrendously expensive mobile telephone bill one evening speaking with me. Alastair talked about his surprise that I had not known about the movie, wondering if I was upset. I said no. Everyone experiences an outbreak differently, even when present at the same time. I felt that the contributors to the film were welcome to whatever echo my participation in Nigeria left in their larger impression of what had happened. In my mind, he was not playing me, he was playing whatever influence by me was perceived by the survivors of the outbreak that had something to do with the film. I have not seen the movie nor read the script. I know nothing more of it than the brief, pleasant telephone conversation with Alastair while he was filming in Lagos. If this differs from that depiction, mine, like all of this writing is a very narrow, personal view.

On the night that I had arrived in Lagos I had a late supper with three people pivotal to my experience there. Kamal Ait-Ikhlef is a WHO logistician with extensive field experience in emergency response. He had arrived a few days before me and begun to work with Nigerian decontamination personnel on safe burial practice and assessment of the clinical center that had received the EVD patient, First Consultants' Hospital. The hospital had been closed and its leadership was eager to reopen. Dr. Emmanuel Musa was the Disease Prevention and Control (DPC) director at the WHO country office for Nigeria. That office is one of the largest of WHO's more than 150 country offices. A Nigerian, Musa, as he is called routinely, managed disease outbreak issues in Nigeria to include cholera. Professor Abdulsalami Nasidi directs the Nigerian Centre for Disease Control (NCDC). Professor Nasidi is an experienced virologist with many contacts in the global special pathogens community. When I arrived, Professor Nasidi was the lead for the emergency response team, supported by Musa.

The drive into Lagos from the airport was a bit overwhelming. I have friends who really like Lagos. The massive expanse of neighborhoods reminded me of New York City. Some were contemporary while others stretched with shanties across floating docks and piers as several waterways meander through Lagos. It was both more affluent and poorer than other large urban places I recently had been. I began to understand the angst at headquarters that pushed me to Lagos so quickly. Fortunately, the hotel was small. When Kamal, Musa, and the professor returned late that night, we grabbed an outside table and ate in dim light. I ordered the pepper pot soup. I already knew and really liked Kamal from Geneva. I never had the chance to ask Musa and Professor Nasidi, but I think that my dinner selection made a difference in how we started with each other. Pepper pot soup is a topic. In Kenema, my local colleagues told me that pepper pot soup was their creation and the best example. Musa and Professor Nasidi assured me that that was the wrong view; Nigeria was the founding nation for pepper pot soup. Indeed, it was different in Lagos than I previously had had, much hotter. It was really good, but hot. Maybe it was that I kept eating it, even though it made tears stream down my face, which helped our relationships work.

The next morning, I went to a public health building downtown with the group where a makeshift Emergency Operations Center (EOC) had been established. State and federal officials with WHO and U.S. CDC counterparts already had organized into Epidemiology/ Contact Tracing, Health Promotion, Ports of Entry and Case Management teams. No Nigerians were yet known to be infected by the traveler. With the help of Dr. Frank Mahoney from U.S. CDC and Ugandan WHO epidemiologist Charles Okot deployed by WHO, the epidemiology team seemed to be building an appreciation of the many people who might have been exposed to the Ebola virus. They had thirty-nine contacts listed at that point based on an exposure period of

July 20 to 23. It was July 29, nine days after the first potential exposures in Nigeria. I did not know much about the index case in Lagos when I arrived and until then had thought that we were much closer to when the case was identified. Most EVD patients begin experiencing their symptoms in earnest eight to ten days after exposure. I was expecting cases, if there were going to be cases, any moment. Kamal already had started training a decontamination team and was assisting with an assessment of First Consultants Hospital, the private hospital where the patient had received treatment. Ultimately, most of the EVD cases would happen in those healthcare workers and their contacts.

Within hours on my first full day, I was in a vehicle and met Frank and a couple of the epidemiology team members at the Lagos airport. Having begun the contact tracing among the healthcare workers, they were starting to scope the out of hospital contacts and were having difficulty with connecting with airport workers who had assisted the patient from the aircraft when he arrived from Freetown. One of them was thought to be sick based upon rumors by colleagues. The sudden transposition from the busy EOC to the back gates of the airport after being directed to several different locations, a quiet place where we were not invited, was a rapid change of pace. Our Nigerian colleagues began the conversation with the airport staff. Frank, experienced with polio-related work in Nigeria, participated. Two airport staff were of interest. One was an outspoken, more senior staff member who consented quickly to a conversation and having her temperature checked. The other was a younger staff member who was fearful and not interested in being interviewed. Ultimately, the more experienced staff member was the one successful in getting the colleague to participate, though the interview was tense. Most of the other airport staff members did not want to be anywhere near us. The epidemiology team was trying to conduct their simple intake and monitoring interviews. Who are you and how can we find you? Who is at home with you? How do you feel? If you do not feel well, what is wrong? Have you had a fever, vomiting, or diarrhea? What is your temperature now? Where is the best place to speak with you tomorrow? Both of the staff members had a history of mild symptoms and needed to be screened for the virus. We had come with an ambulance, which probably contributed to lack of interest in speaking with us. Isolation rooms or a process to intake suspected cases had not yet been established in Lagos. Nonetheless, we moved both persons in ambulance to the anticipated isolation site, Yaba Mainland Hospital. It is a small, district-level hospital in an urban area. Like the Lakka location outside Freetown, it was chosen by Lagos State to host EVD patients because it had tuberculosis and HIV programs.

Several challenges in case management became readily apparent. In fairness, they were very typical challenges at the beginning of an outbreak and the Nigerians had cogently assembled central governance of the response team quickly. While the Lagos University Teaching Hospital (LUTH) had some molecular testing capacity and had made the initial EVD diagnosis on the index patient, no one was ready for ad hoc, let alone systematic, collection and processing of EVD samples in the context of real time suspect case assessment. There was no physical infrastructure fully designated or prepared with human, equipment or consumable resources to manage a suspect or confirmed case. There were no clear administrative mechanisms for the provisioning and maintenance of these nor for the care and feeding of identified suspect or confirmed cases. Kamal was building and training a decontamination team, but it was the only decontamination team, so dealing with re-opening public and private venues where suspect and confirmed cases had dwelled as well as recycling ambulances was going to be a challenge. The private ambulance crews had not yet been trained and were suspicious of the process and their safety. No patient care or IPC practice at any stage had been defined. Nigerian physicians were on strike and had been so for more than three months.

With these two cases under investigation from the airport—even I was hesitant to call them suspect cases as their symptom and fever histories were soft, though I wanted to test them and also drill the processes to see from where we were starting—there were immediate and short term needs, let alone medium and long-term needs. We had collected some basic blood draw supplies from the laboratory at LUTH on our way to the airport. In the absence of a Nigerian clinician and with the approval of the Nigerian authorities, I drew blood samples from the patients and interviewed them again while they were in the ambulance. I had some local currency and the ambulance driver had gotten lunch for them on the way to the site. Fed, removed from the stress at their work site and the shock of our arrival, the interviews improved, and I was a bit less concerned that they were ill. We took some time to tour Yaba, consider our isolation options, and observe them over a few hours. On repeat examination neither of them was febrile, we had observed no vomiting or diarrhea and Yaba was in no fit state for its first EVD-related patients. Both of the airport staff had become increasingly motivated to participate in the home-based contact monitoring process with the epidemiology team. After many hours, the response team chose to send them to home isolation and continued monitoring. We returned to the EOC. The episode provided an extremely useful baseline assessment.

Two days later, we admitted our first true suspect case, Dr. Ada Iganoh. She has published a retrospective of that experience in the February 2015 issue of the *American Journal of Tropical Medicine and Hygiene*. I had expected to see cases before that and indeed the patients were hesitant to report for care, having the natural reaction that, "Just because I feel ill today does not mean that it is bad, going to keep going," nothing other than the usual feeling off tempo when mildly ill. We learned later that the very hard working contact tracers and monitors were screening the contact responses and not engaging the case management team perhaps as often as they might, a common and probably natural behavior everywhere I have seen this work… do you really feel like you are not well or do you just not feel yourself, or maybe you should recheck your temperature because the last one might be wrong…. They were empathizing with the contacts. Regardless, before Ada arrived, my behavior was split.

On one hand, I appreciated the systems gaps should an EVD patient be identified. The two days were filled with meetings and site surveys with each of the committee groups, particularly for case management. The contact count had doubled. Frank was stalwart in trying to fill the need for developing standard operating procedures for everyone involved. Our exercise with the two airport staff helped elucidate some of those needs. At Yaba, we identified two rooms for immediate conversion for patient isolation. Enlarging the focus beyond the simple physical requirements to the actual health system that needs to be in place was difficult. In two days, the two rooms went from being ready enough and available to me, to being declared not ready, to being placed under contracts for renovation and out of my reach. At the same time, I was preaching on the challenges of scale. If you are going to have a case from local transmission from that sentinel case, you are going to have cases, plural. The need will not be one to two beds, but eight to ten beds and in one to two weeks thirty beds. The response team and local government initiated a contracting process quickly, though steered away from simpler tent-based solutions that allow rapid expansion. UNICEF and other agencies were becoming more involved. We were starting to look more broadly at other EVD importation risks such as mass gatherings and we assessed one of the common Christian pilgrimage sites in Lagos for people from all across West Africa. There were revelations about how deceased Nigerians and their family members from abroad were brought into the country for burial. I raised issues around healthcare worker compensation and hedging against the catastrophe we experienced in Kenema when safe and effective care becomes impossible to practice due to insufficient human investment for staffing.

On the other hand, I still was focused on my two previous failed attempts to get to Liberia. The large gap in West Africa, a more diversified and sourced foreign medical team response in these countries with thinly sourced and fragile health systems, was not yet occurring. Samaritan's Purse, the only group to respond initially for EVD care provision when it became clear that MSF already was doing all that it could, which was a lot, still had not received technical assistance, to my knowledge. Liberia already had a large and was about to have an even more extraordinary EVD case burden. So, while I scrambled with everyone else in Lagos, I viewed Lagos as better prepared and resourced, extremely lucky to date without apparent cases and I wanted to be in Liberia. I pestered Geneva by e-mail and telephone in between meetings. WHO headquarters asked me to be patient in Lagos for a little longer. It was my third strike in getting to Liberia. Soon afterward I would watch short, televised footage of the extensive precautions taken for the medevac of one of their expatriate clinical leaders, Dr. Kent Brantly. I found it fascinating on many levels. Until then I had no faith that I would undergo medevac if ill while deployed. And, while Dr. Brantly was being rolled in his bubble with everyone on the outside of this completely protective apparatus wearing full PPE with positive pressure mask equipment, I was taking blood from a suspect case in the back of an ambulance while wearing gloves, a mask, and goggles.

Then, on July 31, Dr. Iganoh arrived in Yaba. She looked sick. We had nowhere to put her. I made liberal use of the ambulance. The two rooms that were to be converted for this purpose were overwhelmed in construction. An ambitious plan to convert a structure for an eight to twelve bed sentinel isolation ward was not yet underway and would not be complete or available while I was in Nigeria. There was an old, empty building in the middle of the Yaba compound. It had two small, simple wards and an office in the middle. It had been an isolation ward for multi-drug resistant tuberculosis (MDR-TB) before a newer isolation compound had been built on the grounds. The building had plumbing and electrical issues, was filthy, filled with old ward equipment but had the best virtues possible under the circumstances. It was available. It was separate from any other in progress activity of the hospital. We immediately set to emptying and cleaning that building. Dr. Iganoh took residence that night. She entered the ward on the right. It became the women's ward. When men eventually arrived ill, they entered the ward on the left. We used the office in the middle for staging and coordination. It resulted in a very awkward IPC practice for donning, doffing, transitions, patient interactions.

While I continued to try and assist response team activity in the EOC and elsewhere, most of my time and effort focused on Yaba once we had patients. Kamal usually was scrambling with the decontamination team during the day, and I would see him and get his much-appreciated help mixing chlorine solution and with other logistics needs each night. Eventually he and I got into trouble with the U.N. country team. We were staying at the hospital until after midnight. According to security doctrine at the time, we were supposed to have been leaving the hospital before sunset. Nighttime movement required a heavily armed police escort. After continuing to ignore these requirements, we were put on notice and threatened with the loss of movement privileges. They actually remained quite accommodating. But, it did mean over time pre-midnight exits from Yaba and so longer periods not being present with the patients.

Every day over the next week we accumulated patients, most of them from the hospital where the first patient was treated. Eventually, I was able to set up a deceivingly organized-looking triage process that allowed us to recycle ambulances (empty and decontaminate them) more quickly. The two isolation rooms that defied earlier preparation finally were available. While they were located across several ground hazards and a walk from the makeshift EVD care center, it allowed better separation of suspect and confirmed cases. Those hazards ultimately would leave their marks on Kamal's arm and my leg, scars from falling into poorly marked or covered ditches.

By the end of the first week of patient care, a couple of very dedicated nurses and hygienists became available to the process. I was conscious of the unorthodox, hazardous layout of the care center and incomplete resourcing. We started slowly with on-site training and observation, slow indoctrination and limited activities. Early in the second week, physician interest started to occur. Dr. Bowale Abimbola, the lead medical officer for the Yaba Mainland Hospital MDR-TB program committed to the EVD care center. Soon, some outstanding internal medicine and surgery house officers joined the effort including Drs. Akinbode Ebemi, Dawodu, Umenze, Opawuye, and Eboh. I took the same approach to orientation with all of them. We ultimately adopted it more formally later along with a brief U.S. CDC-led IPC classroom orientation when Dr. Chima Ohuabunwo successfully recruited more staff in the area, as resources and space became more conducive. Despite these early, crude layout and IPC processes that my MSF colleagues later quite appropriately characterized as horrific, we did not experience any infections of staff at the EVD care center there.

The Nigerian patients with EVD were similar clinically to others I had seen, though all were adults, most with higher education and relative affluence. That many of them were practicing clinical trainees or nurses brought an interesting dynamic. When I was a house officer (specialty trainee), I was sure that I knew what really was going on with a patient's care. Sometimes I actually did. These young men and women were no different. They clearly were bright. The combination of their knowing that they were right coupled with being very sick and so not perceiving reality in quite the same way would have been amusing if not focused on their suffering severe sepsis and being very much at risk. I tend to like my patients, and these were easy to like.

Most of them suffered a febrile, high-volume diarrheal syndrome. As in Guinea and Sierra Leone, older patients with likely co-morbidities such as diabetes or heart disease demonstrated primarily or also with an encephalopathy. As in the other locations, I only occasionally saw heavy bleeding, while hiccups were common when patients were behind in taking fluids and small joint pain was typical in recovering patients. Pregnancy and EVD continued to be a tragic combination. My primary strategy remained volume and electrolyte repletion with oral rehydration salts, empiric therapy for malaria, advancing diet, mindfulness of other syndromes and when needed parenteral (intravenous, IV) fluids and electrolytes. Until later in my time there, when additional staff were participating, I had many of the same challenges in safe and effective care present in Kenema—balancing risks: benefits when an IV line could not be maintained, decontamination and doffing, time with the patients. While plumbing and electrical service improved while I was there, initially keeping spaces reasonably clean and doing anything at night safely was problematic, especially placing IV access. The separated suspect case rooms posed additional patient monitoring and intervention challenges, especially for the nurse and hygienist tending to patient needs overnight. As in Guinea and Sierra Leone, we relied on less ill patients to assist.

In this predominantly healthcare worker outbreak, of those contacts who became ill, most had Ebola virus disease. Communities suffering Ebola virus disease outbreaks have little tolerance for people who are bleeding from completely unrelated reasons. Fear can be intense. Women with maternal hemorrhage, victims of motor vehicle accidents or other trauma may be abandoned to EVD care centers or simply left for dead. Given the limited space and sparse resources available for use at Yaba, we were very fortunate that this phenomenon was surprisingly limited in Lagos. One afternoon shortly after I had visited the patients and doffed PPE, someone came running to the ward and said that the emergency department had an Ebola virus disease patient. I walked across the compound and saw a woman sitting on the ground just outside of the door to the room used as an emergency department. There were people inside looking through the window but otherwise she had been given a large berth. She was dressed in T-shirt, shorts, and flip flops and had blood on her face. I approached to a few feet from her and tried to discern her story. It was slow going. She had epistaxis, a nosebleed. It had been going on for a day. Her live-in boyfriend or husband, I never discerned which, had dropped her at Yaba and left. We spoke in incomplete sentences for some time before she consented to more of a physical exam. I donned mask, gloves, and goggles and was able to do a cursory evaluation. Initially, I was worried that she actually had upper gastrointestinal bleeding that she was perceiving as a nosebleed. In the end, though, it seemed like a nosebleed. She was a young woman and my suspicion for eclampsia, given no visible pregnancy, was low. After some scrambling we managed to get a blood pressure cuff. Her pressure was elevated but within reason for someone both ill with anything and perceiving the fear in those around her at the site. I had trouble getting a history from her of contacts let alone where she actually lived. Assessing her true risk of EVD was a problem. While I did not like the idea of adding to her stigma and stretching our own resources by trying to admit her as a suspect case patient, we really did not know at that point of the outbreak what its nature was, whether it was restricted to the healthcare worker associated community or whether it had branched into the small communities peppering Lagos. With her assent, I obtained a blood sample, completed and then admitted her to a suspect case room. After nose packing, fluids, a meal courtesy of the Yaba hospital director, and some sleep away from the panic, she did quite well. After a couple days, she went home with successive Ebola virus negative blood tests. Suspect case patients require the same isolation infection, prevention, and control practice as confirmed patients, however. So, managing her care over those days in separate buildings from the ward was a challenge. Fortunately, the severe suspect cases experienced in Conakry, and the plethoric case load of Kenema did not appear in Lagos.

Visitors to the EVD care center were rare. A few family members made frequent trips and I always was happy to have them on site. The patients consented to my speaking with them. A couple of family members entered the ward under supervision to visit their relatives. The hospital director, Dr. Gbadamosi, and his never-sleeping environmental health technician usually were on hand when needed. Other than Kamal, Chima and the state case management lead, Dr. Ismail Abdul-Salam, very few response team members would come to the care center. The UNICEF and U.S. CDC teams made an effort to do so, particularly their behavioral health and IPC teams, respectively. The Honorable Jeffrey Hawkins, U.S. Consul General, made a couple of visits and took time to understand the response and risks. The patients' favorite visits, though, were the occasional ones by Kamal and when our other colleague, Dr. Maurizio Barbeschi, took a break from doing Ports of Entry and Mass Gatherings work and passed about books, cheer, and loud Italian scolding of me for spending too much time in PPE. He was working with one of his collaborators on these other issues, a former U.S. Navy physician and professor at Florida International University, Dr. Aileen Marty.

Sometimes visits happened in stealth. One morning I arrived and large, tightly packed, brightly covered care packages were stacked on the ground near the building. They were from the medical director of First Consultants Hospital. We spoke several times on the telephone while I was in Lagos but never met. Danny Glover played him in *93 Days*. The care packages were for his medical staff who had become infected. The patients really appreciated these. Opening them was a bit complex with the packaging and in general I knew that a patient was starting to feel better when I would see his or her package open at the bedside. One day when rounding on the ward, I was chatting with a patient in early recovery from EVD who was experiencing joint pain.

He told me that he was feeling better since using the cream in the care package. Cream? He showed me the tube. It was a non-steroidal anti-inflammatory drug cream. Such creams can be absorbed enough in the body to give systemic levels of the drug, creating the possibility that they can inhibit how platelets work, preventing clotting. In a disease characterized by injury to blood vessel lining and sometimes severe bleeding, that could be a problem. In general, we use acetaminophen or similar medications with EVD patients who have pain rather than NSAID. While no one was visibly hurt by this, especially as in general the patients who used their care package contents already were getting better, I had to have a chat with everyone about how that kind of drug by mouth or in cream and Ebola virus work. Another surprise visit that happened when patients were starting to feel better was the delivery of electronics. In Sierra Leone, I had many patients who busily were sending texts to their friends and family. In Lagos, some of my patients were blogging with mobile devices, including laptop computers. This later would cause much consternation as my MSF colleagues—who by then had started participating in work at the care center—and I struggled with whether there was a way to give them back to the patients after the patients were ready for discharge and decontaminated.

Sometimes visits were less welcome by the hospital staff. The response team and hospital staff were becoming increasingly uncomfortable with congregating local residents and non-involved hospital staff. While I think that their security guards mostly were charged with telling someone if a patient tried to leave the premises, the guards onsite, though they and the observers kept a wide distance from the care center, were concerned. I had heard about this concern in my late-night visits to the EOC but had not really registered it until I had doffed my PPE one night and was approached while walking to our vehicle with Kamal. One man, an engineer associated with the hospital, spoke very loudly and directly. He and the group had several questions. We started a conversation. His questions and those of his associates were cogent and well considered. We discussed what we were doing at the care center, the rights of the patients, and that risks were minimal to the community. The crowd dispersed seemingly very supportive of our efforts. I did not hear anything more about it.

The largest dramas happened outside the care center. One night after having left the hospital and gone to the EOC, I saw Professor Nasidi on the telephone. He gestured to me to go to him. He said, “It’s for you.” It was the Minister of Health. The Minister and professor apparently had been in a conversation about ribavirin, an antiviral medication used by some in the treatment of Lassa Fever virus. Lassa Fever and Ebola viruses are from completely different families of viruses. There is no evidence that ribavirin will help in EVD. It has been looked at for Ebola virus previously. There also are reasons to suspect it might be dangerous. The Minister, an experienced surgeon, knew how to read medical literature and was under a lot of pressure to demonstrate the use of novel approaches in order to increase public confidence. More fundamentally, he probably wanted to find a solution that helped his countrymen in a way that worked quickly and easily. In this same conversation he broached the subject of using IV nanosilver, an experimental drug product. Other therapies actually in pipeline testing and development for EVD that were used more broadly later in the outbreak were not on offer. I was tired and angry at the universe and probably the wrong person at that moment to put into a delicate conversation. In short, I suggested that it was misguided to discuss untested therapies when we all must first do the basics, like getting people involved in the usual tasks—including clinical roles, performing the crucial, simple public health actions, and, of course, not doing harm. A similar conversation had started in Sierra Leone while I was there. My response then was similar and pointed…find me an appropriate local physician who will take responsibility to administer the therapy in a controlled fashion after Nigerian review and I am happy to provide that person technical advice. Show up to the party before talking to me about things that may cause harm. Also, we had several patients who were responding well despite being severely ill. I did not want to sabotage them with an incompletely considered therapeutic intervention. Nor did I want to hurry those doing poorly to an end. The Nigerian Minister was reasonable and responded to the conversation quickly. When I later met him in EOC meetings, he was very engaged.

I empathized with the Minister and other members of the emergency response team trying to do coordination in the event more than I told them, and paradoxically knew a core lesson I wanted to convey but not how to do so gracefully. Navy ships in the Atlantic fleet used to undergo Refresher Training at Naval Station Guantanamo Bay, Cuba (GITMO). Usually done shortly after a shipyard period before re-entering the operational fleet schedule, crews under the watchful eyes of evaluators would take their ships through a variety of exercises in navigation, damage control and other essential functions to safely getting ships from one place to another. Some of these happened aboard the ship, others in training areas. Most Sailors from my era quickly associate the name BUTTERCUP not to the historical sloop but rather the holey, ashore container at GITMO where we all tried to fix low and high-pressure pipe leaks and patch holes in walls while getting more and more covered by the rising water. Shortly after the shipyard period where we had trouble with the maintenance on RAST system for helicopter landing, the *USS Normandy* underwent that training. The ship and crew performed well, and we proceeded home. In order to leave the Naval Station, ships have to head eastward along a southern coast and then turn to the north through a short but relatively narrow channel. As we left GITMO, I was the Sea and Anchor Officer of the Deck. Shortly after leaving the harbor, the Captain had tasks below deck. As we approached our time to turn to the north, the navigator reported not having a visual fix. Near shoal water, areas where the ship risked grounding, navigation was performed with a piloting detail. Sailors on deck continuously sight pre-identified navigational aids such as lighthouses and markers. They use a repeater of the ship's compass located on the sides of the ship's bridge in order to call the compass bearing of the object as seen through an alidade, a visual tool which lays atop the compass repeater. Piloting details would collect these bearings and plot them on the chart every three minutes. Before taking such a watch, officers of the deck, conning officers and navigators carefully reviewed the charts and intended track (course and speed), including what should be the bearings to navigational aids at various points along the track. Even though the piloting team had missed a visual fix, I was comfortable that the ship was in a safe position and moving appropriately to its turning point. The piloting team then stated that no visual fix had been obtained at the subsequent 3-minute interval. We had missed two visual fixes in a row just before we were supposed to make a turn into a narrow channel at a full transit speed. At the same time that the team announced this on the bridge, the navigator also announced that it was time to turn. This is what deck logs read like when reviewing them after ships have run aground and I was acutely aware of this at the time. When the piloting team first called no fix more than three minutes earlier, I had intensified my attention on the navigational aids ashore, felt that we had more time before it was time to turn and selected an adjusted turn bearing off a clearly visible object on land. I declined to turn when the Navigator called it as we were not yet in the channel. Shortly afterwards, I instructed my conning officer to initiate a gentle turn. I also asked that the captain be called to the bridge. As we came out of the turn, before the captain had actually been called, he stepped onto the bridge. He had taken no more than two steps when the navigator declared a fix and reported that we were left of the channel after the turn, and so close to shoal. I ordered a corrective maneuver. Visual fixes now were occurring reliably, and we had kept speed and regained the middle of the channel. Captain DeMasi hauled me to the back of the signal bridge, away from the bridge team. I have never asked Frank how tall he is. At that moment, this former Boatswain's Mate and six-foot five inch-former college football player looked ready to pitch me over the side. I thought that being quickly consumed by sharks in the warm, sunny waters of Cuba might not be such a bad way to end rather than, say, getting stuffed down a gas turbine engine exhaust. Instead of putting an end to me, he said, "Do not do that again." "Yes, Captain." "Chrysler Corporation." "I am sorry, sir?" He talked to me about Lee Iacocca, who had been credited with saving the U.S. auto manufacturer Chrysler… do not focus on the weeds, step back and see the woods. Yes, I had correctly not turned the ship early and it would have grounded had I done so. But the purpose of the ship is to fight and be able to fight when asked and not simply keep pace with an intended track on a chart. I was correct to react to the piloting team challenges and adjust my decision making, but I needed to do it focused on the main objectives. I should have taken off all speed not needed to steer and used the time to reassess the ship's position and the upcoming turn with better data. I should have called the captain earlier. As a response team, while we wanted the right things, we at that moment focused on the weeds rather than the woods.

On another occasion the Yaba hospital director, who was buying the patient's food out of his own pocket, asked me to come to his office.

A contingent of prominent Lagos physicians were visiting him trying to insist that he accept ventilators for the EVD patients. They had been spurred to action because, like Dr. Gbadamosi, they were long-time colleagues and close friends with one of my sickest patients, Dr. Stella Ameyo Adadevoh. She had taught and led several of my patients and the young clinicians who eventually joined the care team. Everyone was deeply impacted by her illness. They expressed concern that she and the other patients receive the highest level of care possible. I empathized and suggested that they join the care team as a few of them were U.S. trained sub-specialists. Four of my Lagos patients died, including Dr. Adadevoh. They would have had trouble surviving even in a referral center critical care special pathogens unit. That said, I was intervening on these patients and very happy to escalate care further if properly staffed to not cause harm to patients or staff. Ventilators, per se, were not the problem. Once we had the conversation about what might be needed to do what they were suggesting, they did not feel that they could commit any of the human resources. Even in the U.S., the well-publicized critical care special pathogen units that received repatriated healthcare workers infected with Ebola virus become overwhelmed with one or two patients. In Lagos, my census was over ten.

Later, one of these sub-specialists, a U.S. trained interventional cardiologist named Dr. Adeyemi (Yemi) Johnson, came to visit me at the care center. He had taken me at my word that I would help them build and execute a critical care program within the EVD care center if they could properly resource it. He had tried to fill a staff roster but could not do so. As our roster for basic care was empty, I was not surprised. He then tried to get clearance from his hospital to participate on shifts in the EVD care center. The hospital said that if he did that, he could not conduct care there until twenty-one days after his last shift. This is a usual public health requirement for returning healthcare workers. It probably was all the more prudent given the situation in Yaba at the time. Dr. Johnson was filled with angst. He was either the only or one of the few interventional cardiologists available in Lagos at the time. For me the choice was simple. As shocking as an EVD outbreak can be, at that moment, acute cardiovascular disease had a much larger case burden and he had to stay where he was.

Yemi was not the only one with angst. Many people in the health and emergency communities in Lagos had deep feelings about the outbreak and its response. There was a constant push and pull between authorities at every level and every agency though generally the groups seemed to be able to work together. Some internationally recognized Nigerian experts on IPC and other issues were noticeably absent. Others were noticeably present. It was a public dynamic not unlike what I later watched from afar in Dallas when that city experienced its micro-outbreak.

On one afternoon when I finally had pieced together an assessment and intake process, I had several contacts present to be evaluated. A bench was at one edge of the triage, phlebotomy, and intake area. One contact was sitting on one edge of the bench and six feet away two brothers, secondary contacts who lived together and traveled to Yaba together, were sitting side by side. A well-dressed woman appeared claiming to be a senior official in public health. Without any introduction or questions to the waiting patients, or to me, she started screaming at me that I was putting one of these two young men at risk for EVD and that I needed to move them. When I started to explain that before they ever arrived the concern was moot, she interrupted me and clearly was not going to join the effort and substantively assist. I told her to go away rather than fight her to explain the details while trying to continue the screening. She vented all the way to the capitol, apparently. Neither of the brothers were or became ill. Tempers were high generally, increasingly my own.

I did not begrudge my schedule but I and, I think, Kamal were getting increasingly fatigued. Maurizio took a picture of Kamal one night asleep, slumped in his dining room chair as we had one of our small midnight suppers. In Sierra Leone I had started to have some minor issues with the chlorine. I had developed a short-lived, dry, non-productive (no phlegm) cough. Also, I had started getting skin irritation, a chemical dermatitis, on my wrists, ankles, and other places from repeated chlorine exposure, sometimes chlorine solution trapping when working in or doffing PPE. In Lagos these problems returned and worsened with the omnipresent, necessary chlorine solution. My cough was almost constant and I would have very brief episodes of shortness of breath after decontamination work or other chlorine exposures. The areas with chemical dermatitis always hurt when working, and often when not. More than the discomfort, I was concerned that if my tracheo-bronchitis or lung injury or whatever it was worsened, or if my dermatitis spread and left me with skin breaches on exposed areas, I would not be able to do the needed work. Also, I had injured my left arm doing lifting work in Kenema, chlorine powder containers, bodies, beds. Sometime in the first few days in Lagos I worsened it… cleaning the co-opted ward building, lifting patients, something. The next year under ultrasound after continued pain and the need to lock and compensate my left arm when lifting, my physician would find a scarred distal biceps tendon and muscle.

The physical discomfort was compounded by what my friend Rob Fowler had coined "inequity tension." He was referring to the stark contrast of suffering in well-resourced academic centers in North America after having worked among the tragedy in West Africa. I felt some of this in Lagos. So many people. So many resources. In many ways, though, I was doing the same work that I had done in Kenema. I wanted to be more aggressive, more effective. Eventually, we were a bit more effective as the Nigerian clinical trainees joined the rotations in earnest at the end of the second week of care, enabling us to be more consistently aggressive. Rationally, I know that in a few short weeks, with a lot of help, there was a reasonably effective EVD care center running in Lagos. Nonetheless, this perception of mismatch added to my view. I wanted everything available and interceding faster.

As we slowly increased the intensity of patient care and managed to add some staff without getting anyone infected, the growing focus was on better space where safe and effective care could more easily be applied.

Lagos State University had a history of work in IPC and microbiology. Early in the conversation about where to place patients and when it became clear that the aspirational new ward project at Yaba was slow going, Lagos State suggested that they may have space and interest. After discussing the needs and space, a skeleton team there was assembled. At the end of a night at Yaba, Kamal and I traveled excitedly to Lagos State. They had an excellent space that would have needed very little intervention in order to use it. They had depth in physician and nursing staff. I wanted to move the patients from Yaba immediately. I do not know why, but they never participated in taking patients for care. Later, though, one of their experienced microbiology-practiced physicians joined the EVD care center team, Dr. Mutu. LUTH, where the government diagnostic laboratory was located, never positioned to take cases though it was a source of some of the medical staff that later joined the care center.

For a while we had been eyeing the nicely laid out MDR-TB ward at the Yaba hospital. One of the Federal members of the case management team, Dr. Joshua Obasanya, worked on TB issues for the Ministry of Health. He was aware of a pending initiative to move MDR-TB care to household rather than hospital isolation care. With the additional help of Musa, Dr. William Perea Caro, another friend and colleague from Geneva who joined us, and Dr. Faisal Shuaib, who had assumed management of the EOC from the Federal polio program, that timeline was accelerated, and the MDR-TB ward made available. At about this time, an MSF Spain team arrived, assigned to help EOC efforts. Two of their team members broke away to assist with case management issues, Dr. Carolina Nanclares from MSF Argentina and logistician Paul Jawor. They were appalled with the conditions under which we were operating but understood how it happened in the heat of the onset of the outbreak. They engaged the contractor responsible for the minor, necessary conversions to put the MDR-TB ward to use. With their help, finally, in the third week of patient care, we moved to that ward. Experienced, competent, and caring, Carolina and Paul assisted with the patient transfer and embedded with the care team. They came at just the right moment, as Dan had done in Kenema. For the rest of that week, we integrated and revised our processes, worked with better resources, brought into practice more volunteers, and worked to make the processes independent of any individual, namely me. In short, they were fantastic and invaluable.

In addition to improved patient comfort and hopefully care, the move had other beneficial effects. The new site was more palatable for the increasing number of volunteers Chima was providing. The layout also was more conducive to visitation by families. Suspect and confirmed case placement made much more sense as did all of the associated processes like donning and doffing PPE, laundry, charting, pharmacy, and other preparations before going into and after exiting the high-risk areas. Additionally, the response team itself was more visible at the care site. UNICEF's Behavioral Health team was able to engage the patients. The epidemiology team also started coming to the source of data, the care center. Carolina and I both had noticed that the epidemiology team was working on presumptions about symptom onset and contacts that were different from what we learned over time with the patients. We understood that as the patients realize that they are safe in the care center, as they start to feel better, the information that they provide improves. This is a combination of feeling safe to share the information and feeling less ill and so recalling more of it. We knew, for instance, that the outbreak had not experienced a patient who had become ill more than three weeks after exposure. In fact, the one patient thought to become ill more than twenty-one days was one of ours and she had become ill about when everyone else becomes ill with Ebola virus, less than two weeks after exposure. The patient simply did not trust anyone enough to come forward when first ill, and then did not want to admit that there had been a delay. The MSF Spain team leader, Dr. Theresa Sancristoval, also came to understand the role of an effective care setting to patient trust and so outbreak data. She changed the epidemiology team's practice and started re-interviewing all patients in the visitors' area four days following admission. Line listings, the way that outbreak information is organized to look at both individual cases and their relationships to others, started to undergo significant changes.

We started discharging patients and seeing more EVD-negative suspect cases, signs of a maturing of both the outbreak and the response. On my last day, as I indoctrinated my WHO clinical consultant relief, Dr. Nicola Petrosillo from Rome, and left him in Carolina's capable charge, the attitude in the response team as well as at the care center were significantly improved. Ironically, some of the same challenges in Conakry were present. We had not meaningfully engaged the vigilance for EVD detection and prevention in the larger health system. Much of our recommendations such as contact self-care instructions and other practices I promoted in other countries had not been taken. The progress in team building and response mechanics that happened around and as part of the clinical response, though, were both significant. The state Chairman honored me with a Nigerian traditional outfit, that I wore despite not being able to carry it like a Nigerian, and after a month in Lagos, I left. In addition to the lessons I learned in Guinea and Sierra Leone, I carried another one. Even in well-resourced settings, response is easier and better when prepared and all of the same details apply as when in less-resourced settings. Those still there would have to leverage all of those and other gains a week later in a secondary outbreak in Port Harcourt.

While I was in Lagos, the U.S. Vice Consul, Mr. Jeffrey Hawkins, sent the following message to the U.S. Navy,

> "I am the U.S. Consul General in Lagos, Nigeria, where the U.S. Government is currently working very closely with Nigerian counterparts to prevent the further spread of Ebola Virus Disease here. Through my work with CDC and the Nigerian-led Emergency Operations Center, I have had the distinct honor of meeting and working with CDR David Brett-Major, a Navy physician currently on detachment to the World Health Organization. I understand you are CDR Brett-Major's commander.
>
> "I have been deeply impressed and humbled by CDR Brett-Major's heroism, sense of duty, humanity, and service. For the past few weeks, CDR Brett-Major has served as a physician in Nigeria's only Ebola isolation ward. For much of that period, CDR Brett-Major was the sole medical doctor interacting with and providing oversight for eleven confirmed cases of Ebola, under disturbingly rudimentary conditions. It would be no exaggeration to say that for the last few weeks CDR Brett-Major stood, often nearly alone, between 20 million Lagosians and a massive urban outbreak of Ebola. He did this at considerable personal risk, as the numerous deaths of health care professionals dealing with the outbreak across West Africa readily attest. A volunteer, CDR Brett-Major worked endless days, suited up in hot, clumsy personal protective

equipment, providing medical expertise when Nigerian doctors were too terrified to treat their own patients. At the same time, he provided invaluable counsel to the Nigerian and international staff of the Emergency Operations Center, and personally briefed Nigeria's Minister of Health and other senior officials. He also showed tremendous compassion, and a truly great bedside manner, in dealing with the devastated relations of Ebola victims.

"I am not fully familiar with the Navy awards system, but it seems clear to me that CDR Brett-Major's truly heroic efforts deserve the Navy's recognition. U.S. Navy personnel here at the Consulate have advised me that the Legion of Merit or the Navy and Marine Corps Medal might be appropriate. I would respectfully ask you to consider these or other awards for CDR Brett-Major as appropriate. I am happy to provide language for any award and to seek out an additional statement from another individual if needed. I have not discussed my request with CDR Brett-Major and he does not know that I have reached out to you, although I will inform him.

"I look forward to hearing from you."

Mr. Hawkins' kindness was generous. What I did not realize when alerted to it was that the military's reaction to this note was less generous. In the context of increasing Defense department reticence in the setting of interagency fervor for more involvement, U.S. military medical leadership found this news jarring. It would impact the on-going administrative drama about whether I was to stay assigned to WHO in Geneva.

Ending in Geneva

"Vou-me embora pra Pasárgda."

-Manuel Bandeira in "Vou-me embora pra Pasárgda", *Vou-me embora pra Pasárgda*

"To curb the epidemic, it is imperative that States immediately deploy civilian and military assets with expertise in biohazard containment. I call upon you to dispatch your disaster response teams, backed by the full weight of your logistical capabilities." MSF president Dr. Joanne Liu, U.N. Special Briefing, September 2, 2014

"Ebola cases could reach 1.4 million within 4 months, CDC estimates" *New York Times*, September 23, 2014

"…follow a chart published every few days by the [WHO]… number of new cases detected in West Africa… showed something we hadn't seen in months: a decline in cases reported in Liberia." *NPR*, Michaeleen Ducleff, October 9, 2014

"Texas nurse who had worn protective gear tests positive for Ebola" *CNN*, October 13, 2014

"The U.S. Military's new enemy: Ebola. Operation United Assistance is now underway" *Washington Post*, October 13, 2014

My experience in Lagos, like that in Kenema, was unconstrained. I had for at least part of the time self-decontaminated at night, been whacked in the face with various limbs, and worked in an environment sub-optimally maintained. Shelly and I again relegated me to the basement bathroom and guest room for over two weeks while re-entering the daily routine at home and work. That work routine, however, had changed. I have been struggling with how best to describe my last two months at WHO.

Increased international attention to the epidemic, for some reason a word people were careful not to use, had brought about change. Maybe this was instigated by Nigeria becoming involved and the evacuation of some U.S. and European health workers. WHO headquarters was attempting to matrix its resources for a better coordinated response to the outbreak. It had done something similar but at a smaller scale the previous year when forming its task force for the avian influenza A(H7N9) and Middle East respiratory syndrome coronavirus (MERS-CoV) outbreaks. My friends tell me that this happened during the influenza A(H1N1) pandemic in 2009-10, also. All of the organizational structures had their usual tasks, but many of the people were either pulled or dual hatted to deal with the range of technical issues in the EVD outbreak. At the senior leadership level, three Assistant Director Generals (ADG) were in the mix. While my cluster, Health Security and Environment (HSE), and the Polio,

Emergencies, and Country Collaboration (PEC) clusters had long collaborated on emergency preparedness and response, several EVD-specific roles had been defined. My ADG, Dr. Keiji Fukuda, was assigned the task of helping at risk but not yet affected countries with preparedness activities. The ADG for PEC, Dr. Bruce Aylward, was tasked with the principal response role. Much of his polio disease management machinery was being leveraged in the field. The ADG for Health Systems and Innovation (HIS), Dr. Marie-Paule Kieny, was tasked with the research and development agenda in the outbreak.

Everyone was very busy and most people had strong ideas about what had to be done. Usually, they were able to accommodate each other. What struck me the most, though, was the sheer number of people involved. Until I had left, for the most part it was the usual, core alert and response and other emergency people who were focused on the EVD outbreak. Everything had been done by them for five months while they also tried to continue their actions for H7N9 and MERS-CoV, the persistent issues with cholera and everything else. Now there were augmented staff, consultants, loaned staff from public health agencies, and consulting firm staff everywhere. Entire floors of the main building were either co-opted and under renovation for the response or reshuffled. It was like watching a start-up company trying to spin off from a parent company, sometimes making use of the long-standing divisions and staff, sometimes not.

I kept thinking about what Dan had said when he had arrived in Kenema, "Where is everybody?" Apparently, they were in Geneva. They were starting to aggregate in Accra, Ghana, where the UN Mission for Emergency Ebola Response (UNMEER) was located. I am sure that they were at the Emergency Operations Centers (EOC) at all of the large public health agencies and ministries of health offices around the world. They also were starting to appear in the WHO country offices of the affected countries. Over the next two months, they started moving into the districts as well.

For me this echoed the lessons of scale I had observed elsewhere. Pushing resources from the top requires a lot of congregated resources there and time. Time to pull together, time to build the vehicles to disseminate those resources, time for people to accept them, time to get used to their flowing to where you need them, for performance and for sorting out what that performance is, time to correct. After the emergence of avian influenza A(H5N1), Severe Acute Respiratory Syndrome coronavirus (SARS-CoV) and several filovirus outbreaks, the same forces that pushed the revisions of the International Health Regulations, member states wanted the WHO secretariat to de-centralize its emergency response in favor of the regional offices. As something in between a WHO staff and tourist, it was fascinating for me to watch the Member States be frustrated by the realities of what they had compelled the secretariat to do years ago when vesting more authority in the regions at the expense of headquarters, then fault it for facing the realities of scale while it tried to reverse its power bases in response to new, soft permissions to do what they used to do. Also, I relaxed a bit about the choice my friendly acquaintance Yoti made when aggregating the Sierra Leone WHO response team in north Kailahun rather than Kenema. To his and others' credit, relatively early on he at least had made a choice that concentrated the resources he had available at what he understood to be the area of risk.

For my part, I migrated into two roles. While I advised a little bit for the preparedness activities, I ended up being pulled into managing clinical operations. Patrick Drury, the head of the Global Outbreak Alert and Response Network (GOARN), and Paul Cox, head of the Strategic Health Operations Center (SHOC), asked me to try and do what Rob had done. Tom and Rob had returned to their lives in the U.K. and Canada, respectively, though they remained connected to the work. Over the late spring and summer, while there were gaps that Tom and I felt most acutely, Rob had shaped the deployment schedule remarkably with overlaps of people in most instances so that the clinical consultants were less at-risk and more effective. I wanted to take this another step forward. I started lobbying for a team deployment approach. Instead of trying to send various individuals into various locations forming ad hoc teams on sites, I wanted to bring mixed teams of clinical and IPC focused staff together into Geneva as a deploying team, prepare them, and then send them to a country team to act with the country-level response team in a coordinated way, with clearer rules of engagement regarding risk and objectives that favored longer term improvement in clinical operations in the outbreak and in the country. Through very robust efforts by administrative staff who never will receive any credit, we were able to pilot that concept. I was able to deploy a few teams into the outbreak. The feedback I received from them was positive. I was variably effective in helping the regional and country offices understand the concept. They occasionally tried to create situations where a single individual would be sent, at risk, alone in a setting similar to Kenema or Lagos. For them, I think that they were accustomed to clinical care being a black box that MSF magically managed. However, the piloted teams understood that they were more effective collectively and were able to resist such pressures. They knew that working in teams made it possible to monitor and assess clinical activities at a site, to enter high-risk areas more safely, provide more rounded input to clinical care provisioning groups and better feedback to the management of the response within the country-level response team.

Dr. Cathy Roth, also pulled me into the research agenda work, trying to advance the availability of investigational therapeutics, vaccines, and diagnostics. Mostly, I think that she did this because she liked having someone with her who continued to use a stethoscope and a pipette amongst the sea of diplomats. It afforded me an opportunity to provide feedback about the clinical experience and stay connected with the evolving science. The clinical management team also fed several experts into the process, including Rob, Tom, Dan, Professor Fred Hayden, an experienced clinical virologist from the University of Virginia. We usually were able to reinforce each other. Cathy, like many of my friends, had an extremely busy summer. She led the technical support in Saudi Arabia for the re-escalating MERS-CoV outbreak and then returned to walk into the Ebola responsibilities. Several of my friends were constantly cycling to and from the field for Ebola and other outbreaks, then back into frenetic headquarters activities on return. Mikiko worked another turn in Kenema and Chris, Lina, and Nadia remained engaged there as well.

Ian and his team managed to bring a coalition of agencies together to build and maintain sites for FMT to work. This enabled the Foreign Medical Team (FMT) initiative to grow as non-MSF entities lacked their logistics capabilities and were unaccustomed to establishing Ebola treatment units. This sometimes, like everything else, could not help but be filled with drama. A site would be dedicated for a new EVD care center, then a community would lobby for its move or, ironically, it would be de-selected because of a pending international donation to renovate it for some other use, like sports. Communities are entitled to prioritize their own interests—this simply accentuated the point. At the time, some modeling predictions provided absurdly high estimates of anticipated case counts, particularly in Liberia. Much like the U.S. response in Operation United Assistance, I think that the FMT work served very importantly in restoring public confidence and capacity in non-EVD related health services. Also, it demonstrated a pathway for some clinical management issues to be more broadly operationally considered in future outbreak preparedness and response. There is more work to be done in bringing clinical expertise into the field in these emergencies cogently, safely and effectively. The public health agencies and other usual partners for WHO have not easily leveraged that kind of capacity for some time.

When I initially took on clinical operations, the staff that Rob and Tom had recruited still were in the field. I tried to act as Rob had done so effectively for me and reached out to each of them. As frustrating as it was to be in West Africa and not be able to connect with people in Europe, being in Geneva and feeling responsible for the staff on the ground while not being able to reach them because the universe simply did not want Sierra Leone mobile telephones to work that day was maddening. I quickly had an enormous amount of empathy for what I had put Rob through. Over the experience of WHO clinical consultant deployments in this outbreak, a few people were transported out of country emergently for potential exposures. Two of these happened shortly after I took on clinical operations, Drs. Lewis Rubinson and Ian Crozier. Both of these men have published their experiences in the medical literature. Ian was already in Kenema and Lewis enroute when I returned to Geneva. I spoke with both of them. I warned Lewis that Kenema was a complete mess, and Ian that I agreed with him that it was a complete mess. Despite my report in July to the Minister and WR that the treatment center in Kenema was unsafe and unsustainable, the response team continued to keep it pivotal in its strategy. They may have received different, time-appropriate advice from those that followed me. I could not help but be frustrated, though. I told Lewis, Ian Crozier, and everyone else deployed of the deployment strategy and rules of engagement I was starting with subsequent teams. I tried to push the guidance to the country offices in advance of the teams so that they could be adopted for persons on the ground. Ian Norton and his FMT group had successfully recruited an International Federation of the Red Cross (IFRC) team into a site near Kenema while I was in Lagos. The WHO consultants in Kenema and MSF worked with them to get ready. But the vast majority of the EVD patient burden in the Kenema catchment area persisted at the same district hospital located EVD care center.

A couple of days after I spoke with Ian Crozier, he developed a fever. Dr. Frederique Jacqueroiz, Dan's wife, cared for him onsite and the country team acted quickly to facilitate his medevac. Fortunately, while his clinical course has been complicated for over a year, he is improving, bright, and someone should hire him to do any kind of work he wants to do. A couple of weeks later, Dr. Caroline Cross, the WHO medical director, called me. She had been managing all coordination for medical emergencies among the many people starting then to arrive in the field. Lewis needed to discuss a potential exposure. As he later describes in his paper in the September 2015 issue of the *American Journal of Tropical Medicine and Hygiene,* where Dr. Iganoh published, he did one small task too many at the end of a long session in PPE in the high-risk area. Removing an exposed needle improperly placed by someone else in a sharps container so that the next person would not be injured, he was cut. He did not want to interrupt his work, but he recognized as we spoke what we understood in Geneva. This was a high-risk exposure and it was time for him to go home. Caroline, the staff on the ground, and country office managed his medevac quickly with the U.S. Department of State that managed the air medevac contract. At Lewis' request, he was transferred to the small National Institutes for Health (NIH) special pathogens care unit. Fortunately, he did not become infected.

Tom had since returned to his duties with the British Army. He advised the U.K. Ministry of Defense effort to field an FMT in the Freetown area of Sierra Leone. The British Army has a medical training site outside York designed for acclimatization and practice in a simulated environment. While used mostly for surgical teams headed to the Middle East, it was adapted for preparing an EVD care center. Tom certainly did not need my help in order to guide someone in EVD care, he asked me to come to the training so that the teams could hear what he had been saying from someone else and feel supported by WHO. As a parent and teacher, I completely understood. My children and students alike usually respond more acutely when someone else comes along and delivers the message I had been preaching. I went and was enormously impressed. They had me back for another training round while Tom was deployed with the first team. In the second round, they had incorporated U.K. and Norwegian health ministry staff who were going to populate various NGO clinical operations as well. Every once in a while, hazardous material-dangerous pathogen dogma employed in the training would conflict with messages that I thought the trainees, at least, needed to hear also.

But, overall, I was afforded leeway. Ironically, the largest additional message I pushed at the training and that met the most resistance was a military strategy one. All plans fail in the face of the enemy. To paraphrase General Eisenhower, planning, not plans, are important. Over the course of the year, I received a few messages from the people I trained that once on the ground, they came to understand what I had meant. Some lessons are learned best from experience.

Meanwhile, Vice Consul Hawkin's complimentary message from Lagos was not met well. What I did not know while working in Lagos was just how complicated the Defense department and U.S. interagency conversation had become regarding support in Liberia. I am told that at the moment of this message, the Department of Defense had just said in response to whether it could support direct clinical management of patients in the Ebola virus disease outbreak in West Africa, no. There are many quite reasonable and predictable explanations why the Defense department may not have wanted to do that then. Burgeoning and long-standing security threats at the time requiring continued focus of logistics support as well as force health protection assets would make the case against distracting from that focus by becoming mired in a large public health response. That such investment would be costly in contrast to what had been yet articulated in terms of national security interests probably was true—though, that view at the national security staff level would shift markedly in days. How to deal with volunteerism versus compelled work for what was perceived to be an unusual hazard, Ebola virus, as well as challenges in safe repatriation of the service members were meaty and appropriate lanes of discussion. Part of what was said, however, was that the Defense department lacked sufficient expertise. And, at that moment, the military gets Mr. Hawkins' e-correspondence with a copy to the director of the CDC and endorsement from the in-country CDC lead.

This surprise and frustration caused further administrative delays. While Navy Medicine reviewed what having an officer loaned to an outside organization meant, and discussed whether it still wanted someone at WHO, the end of October became ever closer. I hate surprises. At some level, I understand their reaction. Unfortunately, there also were missteps in the way that the Navy initially established my position, as far as the Office of the Secretary of Defense and the Government of Switzerland were concerned. These obstacles could not be overcome quickly enough to save the position. By the time that Navy Medicine decided to continue my stay, it was no longer possible.

On October 31, 2014, my term employment as a WHO medical officer ended. Shelly, the girls and I transitioned back to life in the US. I provided some technical advice regarding Ebola and related issues afterwards. However, the Defense department's role evolved without me in the form of Operation United Assistance in Liberia.

Navy, health security, and insider politics

"The only shots that count are the shots that hit."

-CAPT Harry Baldridge quoting President Theodore Roosevelt, "Sims—The Iconoclast", *Proceedings,* February, 1937

“Military names 5 U.S. bases for troop Ebola quarantines” *CBS News*, Associated Press, November 7, 2014

“Study of experimental Ebola drug ZMapp could start next month” *Wall Street Journal*, January 16, 2016

“The International Health Regulations (2005) Emergency Committee regarding Ebola virus disease (EVD) in West Africa met for a ninth time on 29 March. On the basis of the Committee’s advice and her own assessment of the situation, the WHO Director-General declared the end of the Public Health Emergency of International Concern regarding the Ebola virus disease outbreak in West Africa... [in addition to Guinea, Liberia and Sierra Leone, four countries] (Italy, Mali, Nigeria, Senegal, Spain, the United Kingdom, and the United States of America) have previously reported a case or cases imported from a country with widespread and intense transmission.” WHO Ebola Situation Report, March 30, 2016

So far, I have tried to tell the story of my interaction with the Ebola virus disease epidemic in 2014 linearly, in the sense of my broadening experience in successively affected countries and the global effort. A mostly unaddressed recurrent theme of my experiences, however, has been not that of the epidemic itself, the communities involved, response partners, the WHO, nor of a clinician or tropical public health professional, but that of a naval officer. There remained a sometimes quiet, sometimes very noisy tension between my status as a commander in the U.S. Navy Medical Corps and my work in both Geneva and affected countries. Like the rest of this book, I describe it with intrinsic biases and those others involved may view it differently.

The impact of communications in any organization is dependent upon timing. The consequences of those about my deployment to Nigeria were final. Many ironies were at play. Nigeria was my third such deployment. Each time I deployed, in addition to alerting my chain of command I always sent a courtesy alert to the military group in the U.S. Embassy in each country. In Kenema, Sierra Leone, I worked at a site supported with long term diagnostic laboratory investment by the U.S. Army Research Institute of Infectious Diseases and the Defense Threat Reduction Agency (DTRA). DTRA is a significant funder of discretionary health security activities at WHO as well as the CDC. Mere weeks after my experience in Nigeria closed, the cases in Dallas prompted U.S. Northern Command to commission a military rapid response team for potential use across the country if needed, led by my colleague, U.S. Navy Commander Dr. James Lawler, who had followed me in Guinea. Within weeks of that, the Naval Medical Research Center's deployable laboratories were in Liberia conducting diagnostics and initiating the Ministry of Health's capacity to do so, in advance of Operation United Assistance, facilitated with its long-term investment in health partnership through the Accra, Ghana detachment of the U.S. Naval Medical Research Unit No. 3, Cairo, Egypt. I cannot think of a single preventative, diagnostic or therapeutic medical countermeasure targeting the Ebola virus fielded in the Ebola epidemic that was not either a direct or indirect product of the U.S. military's acquisition and medical research and development enterprises.

For me, the best explanation for these inconsistencies is that the military does not know what it wants from global health security work. Ironically, health security is in both the national and maritime strategies, particularly in the context of stability operations. While I am certain that my colleagues at the Pentagon understand the greater good of better global health, the agency itself coming to terms with its niche strategic goals is quite another thing. The White House in 2014 named the Secretary of Defense along with the Secretaries of State and Health and Human Services as responsible for execution of the Global Health Security Agenda. This agenda is designed to organize U.S. and partner actions for better health security in countries that pose pandemic risks, and so globally. Being named as responsible, however, did not result in any rapid, comprehensive understanding. Some of this is because the external view from other U.S. Government agencies is confused about the Defense department's role. There is little supportive external pressure to conform to a helpful unified strategy, rather what exists is competitive pressure for the Defense department to relinquish funding without acknowledging the existence of long-term equities. The Departments of State and Health and Human Services (HHS) have health, health security, health diplomacy, and diplomacy written in their main work lanes. They have a general view of what they want to do, but difficulty other than in ad hoc terms understanding how the Defense department fits within their requirements and goals over time.

Internally, the Defense department landscape is equally myriad. There are acquisition groups that are interested in hardware, laboratory tests, medications and vaccines, and surveillance data that can be bought through focused investments, to include against chemical, biologic, radiologic and nuclear threats. There are healthcare provisioning groups that think about health diplomacy as just-in-time clinics after an earthquake or one-time visits to remote villages. Those managing healthcare services also have to preserve their resources for increasingly challenging care delivery obligations at home and abroad. There are research and development groups that work to advance science and knowledge, product development for the laboratory and pharmacy such as vaccines. There are data collectors and information brokers. There are geographically focused interests. No one entity within the military has the mix of human talent, technical and fiscal resources, access and mandate to work in isolation broadly toward health security consistent with short- and long-term national security needs. As a physician-scientist, I love this for short term projects. If I have an interesting idea and the first group hates it, I have a fair chance of finding it a home and funding elsewhere. For operations or long-term projects, this becomes very tricky. From a systems perspective, maybe fragmented sourcing and strategy for health security works as I must achieve consensus among a mix of stakeholders before I get too much funding.

Dr. Tony Mounts, a senior CDC physician who worked at WHO Geneva when I did, invited me to supper once. At his dining room table, I did a spectacular job of mirroring this Defense department confusion in response to a question from him. Tony probably intended to ask me something very simple, as in, "What do you personally want to get from your time at WHO, and I how can I help you?" Tony has a great history of missionary work—the kind of work in country over time embedded with communities rather than "jump in/ jump out" medicine—in addition to his public health activities, and I thought that contrast with my military background might be hidden in his question. "What do you mean, 'Why am I here?' Longitudinal health diplomacy with science was either born, or if not born institutionalized, in the military during World War II. The overseas laboratories in the military are the cholera and typhoid commissions of the 1940s. They represent host capacity building, long-term health and threat surveillance and countermeasure product development platforms. We are older in this business of tropical public health than anybody else." My response was defensive, out-of-context, and not my finest moment.

The more that I thought about Tony's question, the more difficulty I had answering it consistently even for myself. I was sent to WHO by the Navy. My first choice, working in the Army-led HIV vaccine research program was deferred by the Navy. That happened even though the Army and the Navy entered into a dedicated Memorandum of Understanding to make that happen. The WHO assignment had been filled by three Navy officers before me. The first was a preventive medicine officer. The next two were infectious diseases sub-specialists as I am. The Army over the years had declined to support placing an officer in Geneva. While my predecessor, Captain Matt Lim, was in the assignment, he was, to my understanding a bright and productive member of the WHO team. As he was readying to leave, however, there was some doubt in the Navy as to whether the billet would be continued. For some reason, they did continue it. There was not a clear pandemic threat against which this assignment was done. There was not a WHO program per se that had to be managed by a Defense department official in the way that CDC officials support their counterpart programs in explicit ways such as against polio, influenza, viral hepatitis, HIV or malaria. I think that the long-term view of the Defense department sponsor for my assignment was that eventually a seconded Defense department official would be critical to joint management of such a program around emerging threats. But that long-view was not paired with any workforce strategy to support it. The chaotic nature of the Navy position at WHO and how I came to fill it was emblematic of the larger questions.

From the WHO side, like any large bureaucracy, it has little room in its budget for discretionary, new problems or entrepreneurial activities. The Health Security and Environment Cluster to which I was assigned received discretionary monies from the Defense department for health security-related projects executed with interested Member States. It may be that in the long view WHO thought that that relationship would bear fruit. Functionally, each of the seconded Defense department officials, U.S. Navy officers, interacted quite differently within WHO. Other than the last three of us being so similar in clinical profiles, if you had us in a room and asked what we did within the Organization, you would hear quite different answers as access and utility within WHO or any setting is so personality dependent. I had had several years of international operational, educational, capacity building, and public health response experience prior to the assignment. I imagine my predecessors had a mix of that as well. None of that, though, suggests a long view. The military health system research enterprise comprising principally Army and Navy assets has laboratories in Africa, Asia, and South America. Several of them serve as WHO network referral laboratories. However, those kinds of relationships are built locally and reinforced by science performance. One aspect of being from the Navy rather than CDC within WHO was that as I was not placed there in the context of a joint program, I was free labor in the truest sense. WHO could do almost anything they wanted with me in the context of health security. Who does not like free labor? Also, when my WHO leadership was alright with my doing it, I occasionally was a useful touch point for State, HHS, and the various stakeholders in the Defense department as I was not naturally part of the push and pulls between them on health security issues.

Despite all of this uncertainty, with my vantage at WHO, there were many times that I probably had a better view of who was trying to fund and execute what in global health and health security among the U.S. agencies than anyone in the U.S. Government. All of the technical leaders in these agencies knew that I was in Geneva and available to connect the dot-line diagrams with them. Frankly, I thought it in the best interest of both the taxpayer and WHO to undertake that. However, my counterparts back in Washington and elsewhere probably were never quite sure whether a quiet Navy, Defense, WHO, or other allegiance in me would complicate their goals politically or operationally. Only in brief interactions did anyone in the U.S. Government engage my viewpoint, usually from agencies other than the Defense department. This continued as the Global Health Security Agenda was announced in 2014, about which I have mixed feelings. Generally, it seems a good idea. At its beginning, like other good ideas, it was shoved into diplomatic correspondence and business practices of convenience. It is professed to be about holistic health security, better partner country health and all hazard preparedness and response. However, it is very proscriptive in somewhat narrow technical objectives that avoid broader country-level risk assessment, characterization, and autonomy in priorities. It was introduced so forcefully in the international health community that active development projects I was building with partnering donor and in need Member States disappeared because of everyone's internal clamoring to be seen as part of a Global Health Security Agenda action package with the U.S. Somewhat like a labor movement problem, I foresaw a situation where in-need countries have even less self-determination in a setting where donor countries essentially have organized and constrained the kinds of support available anywhere. These views did not make me popular on interagency telephone conferences. However, the agenda is an organizing force in a security space that I have admitted is chaotic. General Norman Schwarzkopf, the famous commander in Operation Desert Storm in Iraq, used to say that with change, organizations will "form, storm, norm, and then perform." Their constituent parts, sometimes simultaneously, come together, fight internally for their natural or sought after places, consciously or unconsciously develop practices to be able to function together, and finally start to perform their tasks and produce outcomes. In fairness, I have only seen the forces trying to implement the Global Health Security Agenda in the form and storm phases.

These efforts focus on development of capacities and long-term function rather than steps to take in an emergency response. It was fueled most recently by the avian influenza A(H7N9), Middle East respiratory syndrome coronavirus (MERS-CoV), and Ebola virus disease outbreaks of 2012 through 2014-5 but not really designed for active emergency management. As West Africa became increasingly impacted by Ebola virus, the same parties within government that were maneuvering with regard to this agenda also were interacting for the Ebola response. This may have helped or hurt the way that these things happened. Some smart graduate student at war college or one of the government or international affairs colleges should do a thesis on that.

My most direct interaction with the drama associated with these issues during the Ebola virus disease epidemic was on the subject of increasing clinical care capacity. During the summer of 2014, when the passionately unaligned and governmental avoidant Médecin Sans Frontières (MSF) made the extraordinary pronouncement that even they thought military run Ebola virus disease care centers were a critical addition to control of the outbreak, they were not alone. WHO was saying this quite bluntly both in countries when engaging the U.S. Agency for International Development (USAID) led Disaster Assistance Response Teams (DART) as well as in discussions at headquarters. The DART response was to offer assistance in building treatment sites for use by other care provisioning entities. WHO already had worked with U.N. partners and others to develop ways to source the construction of care sites and other logistics. What was missing was a sufficient number of well-resourced, well-organized, autonomous care provisioning groups capable of managing severely ill patients. Fortunately for the Defense department, there already was sufficient sensitivity by the rest of the U.S. interagency about who might be seen as pivotal in this response to prevent real pressure to invite or encourage the military to get on the ground and treat patients. No one can mobilize tools and supplies like the Defense department, however, so all were happy to have military transport and engineers on the ground in Liberia. Training courses also were run by the military group with variable but well-intended connections to WHO, MSF, and other response actors that were providing care and had the requisite experience. The Navy already had a relationship with the Liberian Institute of Biomedical Research (LIBR) and had deployed to augment diagnostic testing in country at the behest of the WHO Extremely Dangerous Pathogens Laboratory Network, followed closely by U.S. Army, National Institutes of Health (NIH), and contractor teams. All of that was labeled under Operation United Assistance (OUA) once that operation was started, but the real mission of that enterprise was visibility and logistics.

I was not in Liberia in the outbreak, but I imagine and have been told that having the U.S. military arrive was calming for communities that had experienced instability, interruptions in healthcare services as well as transport of persons and goods, in some instances community quarantines enforced with violence. U.S. ambassadors in the sub-region had been warning of the fall of the affected countries as fragile states because of the epidemic. The arrival of U.S. forces, also conveniently at a point when Ebola was starting to abate, seemed to introduce a stabilizing influence. I am not sure what would have happened if the U.S. military had stood a care center in Liberia. The U.S. Public Health Service staffed a care center near the airport in Monrovia designed to treat ill healthcare workers. Fortunately, a sign of where in the lifecycle of the epidemic they had arrived, their census was filled predominantly by non-Ebola patients. Their presence may have served like the military effort to promote confidence and so the return of healthcare workers to other care settings in the country, helping to facilitate the re-start of health services generally, at some level knowing that a specialized unit was available to returning healthcare workers should they become ill. That was the intent of the United Kingdom Ministry of Defence care center manned near Freetown, Sierra Leone. Guided in part by my friend Tom Fletcher and staffed also with critical care sub-specialists, they offered an advanced level of care. At times, they were busy but overall, they had challenges recruiting patients who could have benefited from the higher level of care. Ultimately, they received permission to assist a neighboring care center run by Save the Children. Cuban and Chinese military medical teams were active in the outbreak by the end of the year, as I am told was a Russian military diagnostic laboratory.

If all of this seems random and ad hoc to the reader, the reader has been paying attention. Much like my personal administrative situation, and despite some very committed and bright people in every agency trying to make things work effectively, the U.S. government responses in terms of interagency coordination in the Ebola epidemic of 2014-5 seemed to happen because they were good ideas at the time and at some level allowed trickier commitments or loss of implementation-mandate territory to be forestalled. From the perspective of the U.S. military, this was in no small part because, just as in broad health security policy, the military was not sure what it wanted. One obvious marker of this was the practice of Controlled Monitoring Areas (CMA), placement of returning forces from Liberia in secured centers with restricted access. Returning troops were quarantined for three weeks on arrival from Liberia despite being monitored closely in country and kept away from the local populace prior to mobilization to return home. Ironically, at these CMA sites, the local presence of well-developed procedures and resources for diagnostic testing or isolation care should someone actually manifest illness was variable. The entire practice was very fortunate that with so many older reservists participating in the operation that they did not have more health challenges. Hindsight has high acuity and so I can rationalize the practice at the very start of the operation. Local and state level responses to healthcare workers returning from Liberia, such as the nurse held in a tent in New Jersey, suggest that many tangible political forces were at play. But the practice of using CMA did not adapt to the evidence that the operation was low-risk as it continued over months. To me, prolonged use of the CMA was a symptom of not understanding special pathogen risk or associated risk management actions as being part of the Defense mission space, and so not having the usual policy and practice mechanisms in place to deal with it in operations.

Two of the larger Defense department stakeholder casualties from the ways the department internally and externally engaged the epidemic were the acquisitions and product development groups. The one entity in the U.S. Government that is very experienced in testing the range of diagnostic, therapeutic, and vaccination products overseas is the joint military health system research and development enterprise. Despite billions of dollars in medical countermeasure investment over the preceding decades, no one was ready doctrinally or practically to field a clinical trial team into West Africa early enough. And it was not apparent that decision-makers understood this to be a core Defense mission for both force health protection and security of the populace.

The evolving interests of CDC and NIH did not assist the internal military debate. Military researchers who tried to engage were stifled from both within and, when trying to explore needs at sites and gain country access, without. These two incredibly important institutions are fundamental globally to public health and science. However, CDC is not resourced or built as a care provisioning or clinical trialing entity and NIH is not experienced or organized in the field for distributed operations in the same ways that the Defense department assets are. Neither of them has substantial experience drawing on non-governmental resources that do these things, either, as their historic, natural partners have been more conventional research and public health implementation entities. Now, at the end of the outbreak, they both are more experienced at least with vaccine efficacy research in these settings than they had been but possibly at a robust cost to their other numerous obligations, and their experience does not necessarily translate into improved functional positioning for trialing novel products in outbreaks in the future. When some NIH colleagues later approached the military health system research and development enterprise to assist in exporting its clinical therapeutics trial into the outbreak, military researchers were poorly footed by then to assist, and the situation on the ground in terms of clinical care was unconstrained and poorly suited to anything short of a significant deployment of resources in order to execute such a trial. One example of what this has meant in the area of therapeutics in particular is that the Defense department investment in favipiravir (an oral anti-viral medication) through Medical Countermeasure Systems was left with a clinical trial for Ebola virus infection performed by non-U.S. actors in Guinea in a way that did not meet Food and Drug Administration (FDA) requirements and so was not useful programmatically. NIH constructed a clever though essentially convenience population trial where whoever appears for care at a referral hospital for Ebola virus disease gets whatever happens to be available at that site and reasonable to use with the data captured prospectively, as the patient receives care. This is in contrast to the classic randomized, placebo-controlled clinical trial where conditions are made equal between two groups, one that receives an experimental therapy and the other something that makes everyone think that that person may have gotten the experimental therapy until what actually happened is revealed. The more remarkable feat by the NIH was to get the FDA comfortable with it, something the French group that worked in Guinea was not able to achieve. The numbers from that study remain very low and diffused across a few different therapies, so licensure of a medication against the Ebola virus is not likely in the near future.

These agencies with scientific capacity all are inextricably linked and critical to each other in the long term. Fighting over policy space and money is tough on any relationship as any siblings who have not liked what a parent wrote in a will can attest. Nonetheless, the first Ebola virus vaccine trialed in Africa predated the epidemic and was performed in Uganda. It was a cooperation between the NIH and Army against a history of Army and CDC cooperation, benefiting from both Army and USAID investment around HIV prevention and care in the country. There are important funding and program implementation bonds across the interagency. After decades of infrastructure and developing partner and host country relationships, no single one of these agencies and their partners would be able to absorb or replace another's workspace in any reasonable period of time. But it is fun for everyone to pretend that they can while maneuvering in the policy and funding space.

Having a capability, though, and knowing what is wanted from it are very different things and this distinction brings me back to Tony's question. This time, what do we want? For me, the strong language around health in the 2010 National Security Strategy created a pivotal moment. It stated:

> "And we recognize economic opportunity as a human right, and are promoting the dignity of all men and women through our support for global health, food security, and cooperatives responses to humanitarian crises… Global cooperation to prevent the spread of pandemic disease can promote public health… We will work with domestic and international partners to protect against biological threats by promoting global health security and reinforcing norms of safe and responsible conduct; obtaining timely and accurate insight on current and emerging risks; taking reasonable steps to reduce the potential for exploitation; expanding our capability to prevent, attribute, and apprehend those who carry out attacks; communicating effectively with all stakeholders; and helping to transform the international dialogue on biological threats."

In the Naval Operations Concept 2010 document that set an implementation plan for the 2007 maritime strategy, while in some ways it limited the applicability and failed to recognize the breadth of medical assets relevant to the strategy, health and medical were cited in the context of humanitarian assistance and disaster relief. It went on to say:

> "Both proactive and reactive HA/DR efforts are undertaken alongside the host nation; other participating nations; multinational, regional, and non-governmental organizations; and in close coordination with counterparts at the Department of State, USAID and other federal agencies."

At the time, I understood these strategy documents to represent an opportunity for Navy Medicine. A first-tier national strategy objective, global health security could be championed by military medical leadership. Military medicine, having the requisite, unique expertise within the department, should and could drive this operational space in addition to its force health protection mission. At the time, I directed an educational program that educated and trained military medical personnel on skills needed for both force health protection and medical stability operation missions outside the United States. The program operated at home and with partner countries in Africa and South America. In response to the strategy documents, I proposed a training and qualification pipeline as well as billet designations in order to construct a workforce development and management base that could meet these strategy objectives. Ideally, workforce for this mission would come from and reinforce science, product development, and force health protection capacity within the department. It was not adopted, probably not substantively vetted. Had such a practice been adopted, how to populate, use, and then employ after medical officers assigned to WHO would have been more cogent. Eventually and from other influences, Navy Medicine adopted a Global Health Engagement office. It may have been constructed with the best of intentions and yet a coordinating office is only as good as the level of clarity present in the organization's related objectives… the organization still must learn what it wants.

Military medicine has little incentive to want something complicated relating to global health. Its leadership almost always is developed from the larger, care provisioning part of the military health system. Faced with one of the largest healthcare systems in the country responsible for nearly ten million beneficiaries, as well as an only recently closed decade-long period filled with severely injured war casualties and medical deployments into the Middle East, a billion-dollar plus surprise pharmacy bill atop the usual costs last year, there is little wonder as to why the focus is elsewhere. If the human talent necessary for the military research and development enterprises were not resident in the military health system, and force health protection not part of the mission so viscerally related to the provision of health care, more people would be making the argument that within the Defense department the entire endeavor should be moved over to acquisitions programming. They would say, "Keep it simple, make all of it about buying stuff and paying someone else to maintain it, possibly to use it." The U.S. and overseas based laboratories, the health research planning and funding, the personnel, all of it could be moved. Such a change would give the Defense department clarity on its role in global health security making it all about building or buying countermeasures and their maintenance and enhancement lifecycles. It would simplify, also, how the military health system wants to perceive humanitarian assistance, just in time, transient application of healthcare delivery resources. But you cannot separate people from their mission, and they are developed within and oriented toward achieving better health outcomes fundamentally. While useful to expose problems and consider program adjustments, such a change would be fraught with hazards.

I retired from the U.S. Navy in the spring, 2016. Now as a pensioner, I have tried to characterize my views—as sometimes I am asked—watching the members of the U.S. interagency continue to form and storm while trying to norm and perform on health security issues, awash in the creative history of recent outbreaks, cyclic affirmations of the importance of health to national security, and waves of sometimes storied, sometimes available repurposed taxpayer money; similarly for the ever-present cycle of secretariat reform within WHO imposed by the Member States and variably touted in the media, a visible reflection of countries' will and its primacy in a member state organization, that sometimes the secretariat is supposed to lead, other times supposed to facilitate, other times supposed to subordinate and act like the omega of the wolf pack, offering itself for devouring by others, its U.S. military-like structure with an astonishingly broad mission set with comparatively few discretionary resources.

From all of this, I have realized that I really do not have one, a view. There is a detachment to having graduated to solid middle-age. Several years ago, I wrote an indignant and sophomoric letter to the American Society of Tropical Medicine and Hygiene, published in that Society's journal. As a tropical public health professional, I was incensed by the convenient wander of terms of art demonstrated by global health, international health and the like, attempting to create wonder, excitement and redirected funding. I perceived them as minimizing the work that I and my betters had done over decades. In these security and health security contexts, however, maybe shifting nomenclature, forcing again new forming and storming, is the correct thing to do. We, not the royal we but the absolute we, still have not demonstrated what we want from health security and national security, otherwise we would have obtained it.

So, maybe continuing to shake non-outcome based organizational and operational structures into new ones through vehicles like the Global Health Security Agenda is healthy, until we know what we want and get it. I probably should have realized when I wrote that letter to the tropical society that what people called the work should be irrelevant, if the outcomes are strong and fundamentally applicable. And if they are, the resources should follow even if so much structure follows financial incentive. Besides, I continue generally in this line of work. As Shelly once observed, the work I like is the privilege of governments and their partners. I remain hypocritically connected to the entire, well-intentioned mess.

Chris Lane recently sent to both me and Mikiko Senga T-shirts. He has returned to Sierra Leone several times in order to assist with the now graying outbreak response. They say “Sierra Leone: Ebola don don”. A few days after he had placed the celebratory clothing in the post, more Ebola virus disease cases were discovered. They or something like them will continue to be there, at home and elsewhere.

I will be just as surprised as everyone else to see what we do about it, each time.

Essays on our ancient relationship with infectious diseases

We are in an abusive relationship with emerging infectious diseases. infectious diseases. We make excuses as to why we should enjoy quiet periods without committing to making the situation better. We tolerate suffering, particularly when it is directed at others. We either wait too long to seek respite when things are bad; or, we see hints of familiar pain, overreact, and make small situations complex. We sometimes are willing to talk to others about it, but we are reticent to overcome inertia and change our habits so that we do not repeatedly experience the same cycles. These essays explore a little bit of our history of fear and dysfunction with emerging infectious diseases and translate some of that history to modern conundrums. They are for the many casual and intense readers who see the news and wonder, really, again?

Learned fear, and a short history of the plagues

The pandemic threat, the suffering of masses by an unseen force is ingrained in our species memory. The roots of plague, pestilence, befalling of suffering are ancient, and not only Christian. The Qur'an refers to many stories about plagues. In Hinduism, plague is mentioned in the Hymns of the Atharvaveda, "Release me from the curse's bond and plague that comes from Varuna," as well as in the Rig Veda.[1] Plague does not seem to be a part of Buddhist ideology,

---

[1] Hymns of the Atharvaveda Book, Hymn 112

which seeks to accept the state of nature and encourages individuals to transcend apparent suffering.[2]

The Bible, in contrast, has at least twenty specific references to plagues.[3] The first such mention is in Exodus, "...If you refuse to let them go, I will plague the whole of your territory with frogs. The Nile shall swarm with them…." It is a verb at its first use, a punishing, willful act upon Pharoah by the Lord of the Universe for not bending to His will, when in fact He set Pharoah's mind against His own will to make an example. There is no escape, all aspects of it are beyond control. The injection of suffering is divine. The last mention is at the end of the Revelation of John, and though a noun, it is given as a threat. "...should anyone add to [the words of prophecy], G_d will add to him the plagues described in this book…," perhaps referring circumspectly to war, famine, death, vengeance of the martyred, and cataclysm of earth and sky, but also more specifically to Death and his wielding of sword, famine, pestilence, and wild beasts, the arrival of an end that cannot be averted.

The earliest roots of the word plague in English are linked to wounds. Broader use as an affliction, a calamity exist from the late 14th century, referring to the Revelation of John and fire, smoke, and brimstone.[4] This reference is forty years after the Black Death was

---

(https://www.hinduwebsite.com/sacredscripts/hinduism/athar/avbook07.asp)

[2] A Buddhist Bible (http://www.sacred-texts.com/bud/bb/index.htm)

[3] **The New English Bible with the Apocrypha, Oxford Study Edition.** Oxford University Press, New York, 1976.

thought to have been introduced by *Yersinia pestis* (the causative agent of plague the disease) infected rats on a merchant ship calling on ports from Crimea to Sicily, causing astonishing mortality stretching across those decades. As notable historians John Garraty and Peter Gay put it, “The shock halted more than two centuries of European demographic and economic growth.”[5]

We are taught to fear plagues by experience, tradition, use of language, dogma and doctrine. We have earned that fear over centuries, just as we have earned the fitful ways that we interact with each other.

---

[4] **The Compact Edition of the Oxford English Dictionary.** Oxford University Press, Glasgow, 1971.

[5] “The State System of the Italian Renaissance”, **The Columbia History of the World.** Harper and Row Publishers, New York, 1981.

What does a healthy relationship look like?

"It's time to close the books on infectious diseases, declare the war against pestilence won, …." William H. Stewart, U.S. Surgeon General, 1967[6]

Communication and honesty

Denial can be helpful. Every time that I go for a hike with my children and watch them strike ahead of me on a difficult trail, or bicycle ride away from me on a path around a bend, I employ it. I could not function as a parent if I did not deny the risk to my children. I use denial each day that I drive in a city and change lanes or hope that cars will stop at a red light, or when entering my credit card and banking information on an internet page. However, as most people experience, denial also is troublesome. Three days remaining before a long paper is due is plenty of time. The bartender is pulling another pint at midnight, but I am sure that I will be fine on my o'dark: thirty run. Filovirus outbreaks have happened in central Africa every three years or so for decades, but that is no reason to think that one will happen again anytime soon.[7,8]

---

[6] As recounted by Michael Specter, *The New Yorker*, January 5th, 2015, https://www.newyorker.com/tech/elements/william-stewart-science-erroneous-quote, acc. June 10th, 2018

[7] Centers for Disease Control and Prevention (CDC), https://www.cdc.gov/vhf/marburg/resources/outbreak-table.html, acc. June 10th, 2018

[8] Centers for Disease Control and Prevention (CDC), https://www.cdc.gov/vhf/ebola/resources/outbreak-table.html, acc. June 10th, 2018

Each of the two years after the West Africa Ebola virus disease epidemic was declared over in 2016 saw notable filovirus outbreaks, Marburg briefly in Uganda in the fall of 2017, and a larger Ebola outbreak in the Democratic Republic of Congo in mid-2018 when for the first time in that country, urban transmission was observed.[9,10] I mentioned these in the introduction to the book. I was in Uganda while they had the Marburg outbreak, quite by accident. I was part of a research team in country to coordinate with a site in western Uganda that I and others developed to be ready to conduct a therapeutic drug trial against filovirus disease (Ebola and Marburg, among others, potentially). While we were waiting in Kampala for meetings and packing to leave for the western district, we were asked to accompany our partners to the national emergency response meeting for the outbreak. We provided some technical support there, and subsequently in the affected villages of Kapchorwa and Kween. While in the health center in Kapchorwa, a young healthcare provider was being interviewed by one of the district level responders. They had cared for a known Marburg patient shortly before that patient had died. A week or so from spending time with the patient, a classic interval for becoming ill with the disease, fever onset. Quite simply, the healthcare

---

[9] World Health Organization (WHO), Disease Outbreak News, October 25th, 2017, http://www.who.int/csr/don/25-october-2017-marburg-uganda/en/, acc. June 10th, 2018

[10] World Health Organization (WHO), Disease Outbreak News, May 13th, 2017, http://www.who.int/csr/don/13-may-2017-ebola-drc/en/, acc. June 10th, 2018

provider was a suspect case for Marburg disease. Uganda is a practiced country when it comes to filoviruses like Ebola and Marburg. And yet, even though I was recognized in the country as being an expert, I could not get the response team particularly concerned about this patient, their risks and the risks to others. Fortunately, the case was mild or did not result in onward close contact with expanding case counts. It might, though, have been disastrous.

Ebola and Marburg viruses are not the only infectious diseases which I have encountered that thrive on denial in real time. Years ago, I ran a training and education program for military tropical medicine. One of my fellow faculty members was with me in Guyana on the northern coast of South America. We worked in a small village afflicted by a surge in malaria cases. We spent a few days there assisting with diagnosis and treatment, as much exposed to the parasite-carrying mosquitos as the villagers. Within a couple of weeks after this, my friend had returned to the United States and developed fatigue and fever. He went to an emergency room in a small military hospital.

He said to the treating physician, "I am a field microbiologist, and I just came back from a mission in a malaria outbreak. I have a fever. Please treat me or test me and treat me for malaria."

"You do not have malaria. We do not have malaria here."

"Right, I know, but I just came from the field, I was diagnosing malaria in people in Guyana, got chewed by mosquitos even with DEET [repellant]. I am sick. Please treat me or test me and treat me."

"You do not have malaria."

Fortunately, this friend called another colleague of mine, who immediately placed a telephone prescription for him for antimalarial therapy at a local pharmacy.

We do not want to believe that certain infectious threats are real and in our midst. We carry baggage about what we must do, or, how we must act in general or with each other if a threat is manifest, and we do not want to face that. In the case of malaria in my friend back from Guyana, perhaps it is co-evolutionary. Malaria is an old disease. Perhaps part of its survival over millennia is its ability to make us unconcerned, promoting apathy. There is early evidence that we think differently when we are infected with parasites.[11] This phenomenon goes beyond parasites. We simply are not ourselves when we are sick. Most experienced physicians and other caregivers will attest that the adage is true that people do not think right when they are sick. Cognitive impairment was very common among my Ebola disease patients, ones I have seen with Lassa Fever, and many other severely ill patients. Maybe all of this happens on a community level as well.

---

[11] Bak J, et al. The Association between Suicide Attempts and *Toxoplasma gondii* Infection. PMID 29397671

Communities experience their members' suffering. And, they have their own communal interests at stake.

The Marburg response team's denial of that suspect case, for instance, is akin to other experiences that I have had when overwhelmed people both subconsciously and consciously recognize that more steps would have to be taken, more energy spent than they want, if they opt to acknowledge the facts before them. Once I answered hospital call for Infectious Diseases in the emergency room for an older, active man with a seemingly sudden, bad pneumonia in both sides of his chest. The gentleman presented ill shortly after the Severe Acute Respiratory Syndrome coronavirus (SARS-CoV) epidemic, at the same time as avian influenza A(H5N1) was causing sporadic clusters of human cases in South-East Asia. For an academic clinician in a US metropolitan referral hospital, his family's interview was suitable for a situational comedy. Every question that I asked which fell into the should-ask-but-do-not-believe-it-necessary category was replied to in the affirmative. Yes, he had just returned from an extended vacation in Asia. Yes, he had traveled through Hong Kong including in hotels suspected of being a part of the recent SARS epidemic. Yes, he had traveled to China and not only completed a Yangtze river cruise, but had long visits with families in villages among chickens capable of having carried H5N1 bird flu. Yes, he had started to feel ill at about the time after his exposures that one might expect for either one of these diseases. And yet, when I did what anyone would have had to do in that setting, which is recommend careful infection prevention and control practice and aggressive medical care; admission to the critical care unit in a room which we had capable of isolating such viruses from other patients; and, pursue laboratory testing for the viruses, I received several incredulous telephone calls from rather high stations in government as well as dismissive ones from local public health personnel. The patient ultimately died without a diagnosis, in an era when we easily could have missed these viruses even if doing focused testing.

Denial is real in emerging infectious diseases risk management. The National Domestic Violence Hotline lists nine signs of an abusive relationship.[12] Two of them are directly related to denial, demeaning communication and denial that what is happening is abuse. Similarly, among signs of a healthy relationship, communication is constructive and honesty is present. Neither can exist when people deny what is happening before them, or what will soon occur. And, cooperative decision making, or even basic decision making, requires it.

What else, then, suggests a healthy relationship? According to the Hotline, respect, trust, equality, mutual choices, economic partnering,

---

[12] The National Domestic Violence Hotline. Relationship spectrum. http://www.thehotline.org/healthy-relationships/relationship-spectrum/, acc. June 10th, 2018

and joint parenting of those under care. Like denial, communication, and honesty, each of them has parallels in the ways we interact with emerging infectious diseases.

Respect, trust, and equality

While some emerging infectious diseases are created by our methods of disease control in both resource-poor and wealthy areas such as the challenges born from antimicrobial resistance, new and re-emerging threats to human health most often emerge from zoonotic events in tropical areas, diseases jumping from wild animals into people, or wild animals into livestock and then into people, directly or by way of an infected vector like a mosquito or food.[13,14] Does this allow an opportunity for respect? Those living on the edge of human communities and the wild surely respect its more immediate dangers, like the bite of a poisonous puff adder snake in Africa or a cobra in Africa or Asia, or the physical challenges of rough landscapes and climates. While the general notion of malaria after working in the jungle, or mortal sepsis following the bite of a Komodo Dragon are part of the social consciousness of some communities, what drives people into these zones are need for food and resources like wood and

---

[13] World Health Organization (WHO). Focus on AMR - evidence, guidelines and publications. http://www.who.int/infection-prevention/publications/focus-amr/en/, acc. June 10th, 2018

[14] Allen T, et al. Global hotspots and correlates of emerging zoonotic diseases. PMID 29066781

minerals, or arable, tillable land. They respect that life is difficult, but not the singular new disease threat. The threat of a sporadic disease pales to their basic survival or growth needs.

Part of this inability to respect disease threats stems from a lack of trust. We learn to trust through repetition. This starts early in our lives. Good parents provide even support and correction regardless of how we act, and so we learn to trust that relationships can last. The many speed cameras on Connecticut Avenue in posh Chevy Chase, Maryland, reliably trigger at 5 mph over the speed limit, and so we learn to trust that the annoyingly slow driver in front of us is just being sensible, and the speeder is either really late or a tourist, and in either case about to bolster city revenue. Sporadic zoonotic crossover events, in contrast, happen sporadically. If they happened enough for us to understand how often they happen we might know enough to stop them. And, even when they happen, even when someone gets infected from a virus that came from somewhere deep in a jungle, whether someone gets sick enough to cause others to get sick, or to present for healthcare, is variable. If someone does get sick badly enough to matter, they might die where they were exposed in a place away from others. If they do not, they may be mildly ill or severe. If severe, in the case of Ebola disease, and near other people, they might infect a couple people or a hundred. And, if many people do get infected from the index case, the first case to get the disease in what might become an outbreak, those people might or might not become ill. Even with

Ebola disease, we are starting to understand that some infections and even limited outbreaks may happen without much impact to people.[15] In this context, the chances for adult learning, for seeing and understanding and trusting that a risk is true and persistent, are fleeting. We do not trust that an outbreak will happen, nor do we trust that it will happen to us.

Something rare, variable, remote, cannot be equal to us, in our thinking. We experience our more urgent realities all of the time, the need to eat, drink, seek shelter, bathe, work and be with others. When measuring any of these against a hypothetical or even known but rare event, they must be greater than disease Z that still is in an unknown place, in an unknown animal, that may or may not interact with us.

Troublesome aspects of relationships between the scared and well-resourced and those that more commonly become afflicted compound this difficulty in appreciating and acting against disease risks.

Mutual choices, economic partnering, and joint parenting

Just as when trying to meet someone at a party or in online dating, a person has to be present with a threat before there can be a risk. Risk

[15] Richardson ET, et al. Minimally Symptomatic Infection in an Ebola 'Hotspot': A Cross-Sectional Serosurvey. PMID 27846221

is the combination of a likelihood and an impact. The more time spent closer to a threat, the more likely it is going to be a problem. And, the setting where most pandemic disease threats are, along margins of human communities and nature or in crowded, impoverished urban settings, the limited nature of resources that those most often exposed have available to endure changes in their health or communities means that relatively small threats can have a large impact. If there is not enough or only just enough wealth to provide the basics of life and community function, there is not enough wealth to invest in managing problems before they occur.

Contrast this with the situation of those who do invest in managing future problems. The gross domestic product of the Democratic Republic of Congo—where both 2016 and 2018-2020 Ebola outbreaks occurred—was roughly 450 US dollars per person in 2016. In that same year, the United States' gross domestic product was well over 57,000 US dollars per person.[16] There is no possible way for people in the DRC and the US to have a balanced relationship involving resources applied to pandemic preparedness. No matter the altruism, the entire public and private marketplace must favor the payer. And while the US has challenges with occasional hantavirus in the southwest, influenza and antimicrobial resistance everywhere, and

---

[16] The World Bank data portal, https://data.worldbank.org/country/, acc. 28 June 2018

even plague, the bulk of experiences with emerging infectious diseases threats is in DRC, not the US.

What must that imbalance feel like, to have an unseen hand drive the choices available in one's own house, and what directions are possible if moving to face them? Is disease Z and its risk management starting to seem like your worst romance?

Relationships with abstractions are challenging. We have a natural way of dealing with this; we personify them, make them as human as we can, infuse persons and things with sentiments so that we can touch how we feel. We love the freedom of getting from place to place whenever we want with our car. We love and name our car. This happens when we hate, also. We focus our frustration of intolerance and fear of genocide as hate of the swastika. We focus our high school insecurity and fear of unpredictability into hate of a taller, better looking, more popular classmate who probably was smart, an athlete, and intolerably nice given the chance. There is no rational measure of degrees. We may exude the same level of angst against both the swastika and the popular one without any insight that this is the case.

We do this with our fear of disease. The disease exists as a person who has it, who must be different, separate, rooted in behavior or status that made them vulnerable, culpable for their affliction, aspects that we decide the person could have controlled, that are far away from who and what and how we are and do what we do, so that we could not possibly be at risk for what we fear. Being separate from these people keeps us separate from the threat, even when those afflicted have little to do with our own risk. **This is a root of stigma.** For me, this is best exemplified by an ancient root, leprosy. We continue to behave like this today. It is part of our relationship story with emerging infectious diseases.

Leprosy, also known as Hansen's Disease, is an infection by a slow growing threat that likes temperatures just below core body temperature.[17] The pathogen, *Mycobacterium leprae*, is thought to infect people via the lungs and mucous membranes, though it does not do so efficiently. It then finds its way to cooler parts of the body, in particular the skin and nerves, especially at the tip of the nose and ears. Depending on an individual's immune response, sometimes it stays very localized, other times it spreads throughout the skin and causes loss of sensation. Without treatment, those severely infected eventually start losing those parts of the body heavily infected, from trauma and other infections. Those most unfortunate appear to have lion-like faces and amputation. They are marked and visible in their affliction. This has made it easier for people to view them as manifestations of their own risk, to hate and fear them.

I used to take physicians training in tropical medicine to a small clinic in Georgetown, Guyana, which served as that country's referral clinic for diagnosis and treatment of *M. leprae* infection. It was a simple place with two treatment rooms and another small room for a laboratory. Patients suspected of having the disease, especially disseminated disease, were tested usually by taking a small razor to the top edge of one of the ear lobes. The tissue is cooler there and it can be a useful place to find *M. leprae* organisms. A very small slit

---

[17] https://www.cdc.gov/leprosy/

allows interstitial fluid to be squeezed onto a glass slide, air dried, then stained and examined under the microscope. For those of us trained in usual techniques in well-resourced places, how effective this can be is surprising. Even though Guyana has a persistent leprosy problem, the total number of cases is small and the most common situation in that clinic is not that a patient asking to be seen has leprosy. In patients with darker complexions, lepromatous lesions can be lighter, have less pigment, than the rest of the skin. This also happens with some very common fungal infections. A young man working in the field with few opportunities to use clean water for hygiene and only a couple sets of clothes might experience significant stigma, shunning, simply because he could do with a change in his daily routine and perhaps an oral antifungal medication for a couple of days. Those experiencing that from their neighbors, or who are afraid of it happening, may seek care for that reason, not leprosy, per se. Leprosy medication is free and provided globally by the World Health Organization. But, learned fear of how the community might react delays and drives pattern of the care seeking. Guyana and some other countries have social assistance programming for those that are identified as infected.

Scrolling through television channels one day I happened upon the movie Braveheart, a scene where the Bruce, a Scottish prince, is speaking with his father in a secluded chamber of his castle. In the movie, the father, Robert the Bruce, had acquired severe leprosy while on one of the crusades to the Middle East. The film's creators used leprosy as a vehicle to force tension between the young Bruce's affinity for the resistance fighter William Wallace, and a responsibility for his father's legacy and realpolitik. The father was forced to remain in the shadows. Despite the fact that the father probably did not actually have leprosy, the film exploited the idea of leprosy—its fear and stigma—because modern audiences still identify with it. It works. How did the idea of leprosy and the plight of life that caused and then is suffered by the leper become so ingrained in even our modern psyche?

For the part of the modern world linked tightly to a Judeo-Christian tradition, it is easy to blame the Bible, or the movie Ben Hur, or other related post-World War II filmography. In their writings, the apostles draw upon lepers to communicate Jesus' radical liberalism against a societal penchant to place the meekest away from those less weak. But, in its telling, even this embracing of lepers reinforced the idea that they needed something spiritually unclean drawn from them. "'...if only you will, you can cleanse me,'" asks a man of Jesus in Luke 5:12-14. Jesus also refers to the man's cleanliness and advises a Judaic rite of purification. Even in the movie Ben Hur, and I refer to the Charleston Heston version, Ben Hur's mother's and sister's leprosy are emblematic of the phase of the movie pervaded by evil, first from Rome and second by Ben Hur's own willful seeking of revenge rather than faithfulness.

Mention of leprosy and lepers in the Old Testament starts in Leviticus. Navigating chapters 13 and 14, in particular, is a heady task as skin diseases and quarantine are laid in serial scenarios, mixing a variety of requirements based on being "ritually clean" or "unclean". To be fair, leprosy is a hard condition to wrap thinking around cause and effect. Latency, how long the offending bacterium sits in the body before a person shows disease, may be very long, in some instances taking years to be visible. And then, either slowly but persistently, or quickly because of a change in the person's overall health, the bacterium sets to work in earnest and shows itself through the person's suffering. The stressed, the undernourished may be most susceptible to the bacterium's work. And, those in poor, crowded settings may be most likely to encounter the bacterium once it is busy in a home, or a community.

And so, the association is made early in this biblical disease. If you are hungry, massed among others, living in squalor with little mobility and you are stricken with leprosy, you are unclean. The more affluent who, in times when life is held with lower value, fortunes rise and fall with less predictability, may already fear the proximity of an impoverished life. They now have spiritual justification for their wellness, for their being less vulnerable and more well. To see the leper before you could evoke thankfulness and charity, or unfortunately fear and righteous pride, distance.

While an old problem, leprosy and fear of it and of those with it is persistent. Exile of cases diagnosed in Hawaii to Kalaupapa continued into the 1960s. And, resettlement of those who lived there in some cases for decades is a startlingly recent problem that carries debate around leprosy's impact on the long term value of the land itself.[18] Louisiana's Carville colony continued to receive patients until 2005, now hosting the National Hansen's Disease Museum.[19] Even in the face of advanced diagnostics and widely available, effective therapy, the disease remains feared. Our enlightenment, though, has difficulties with trust. A second strain of *M. leprae* has been found to infect both armadillos and patients in the United States. And, antimicrobial resistance touches this disease as well.[20] As the disease insidiously evolves, it reinforces the translocated mistrust onto its victims.

---

[18] https://www.theatlantic.com/health/archive/2015/05/when-the-last-patient-dies/394163/

[19] https://www.hrsa.gov/hansens-disease/history.html

[20] https://www.ncbi.nlm.nih.gov/pubmed/30016255

Measles is bad. Vaccines are good.

We will get past the noise around vaccines. We need them. And, those who think we no longer are at risk for the devastating—in some instances society crumbling—predations of measles, mumps, rubella, diphtheria, tetanus, pertussis, *Haemophilus*, polio, rabies, meningococcus, cholera, Ebola, and even still smallpox or its cousins, influenza, and others, simply are either ignoring or unable to understand some of the deepest lessons of history. We need an HIV vaccine, a tuberculosis vaccine, a universal influenza vaccine, and more.

We have much to learn about vaccines and how we employ them, though. The recurrent noise against vaccines offers an important opportunity to think roundly about the patient and community experience with them. In some ways, health system attitudes about vaccines have enabled the radical discourse that seems peaking against such an obvious global public health absolute like Measles Is Bad.

My household is filled with strong vaccine advocates and related professional practice. However, when my wife delivered our children, we could not take them from the hospital without their receiving a hepatitis B vaccine that did not change the vaccine schedule and so they were going to have to get the full series anyway, in a closed healthcare system that knew both our vaccine and even antibody status against Hepatitis B, and where pediatric follow up visits occur at a rate of 100 per cent. When we simply asked the question about why my children were about to receive injections, we were met with shock and aggression. When our eldest child presented for a toddler visit with her pediatrician, the varicella vaccine literally had just flipped from optional to recommended on the American Council of Immunization Practice (ACIP) schedule. She had several shots scheduled, and we conferred with her physician about presenting again in a few months for the new vaccine. Yet, the public health group at the hospital undertook an immediate screening of an affiliated daycare, potentially violated HIPAA procedures while exploring our child's chart specifically, and then ignored the physician: patient discussion that had occurred with their most senior pediatrician. When we have asked basic informed consent related questions regarding an array of newer vaccines, even in instances when the prior version of the vaccine was removed for complications, we have sometimes been met with uninformed practitioners both un-resourced with necessary information to achieve informed assent let alone consent, who were deeply disinterested in and hostile to having adult conversations.

Some of these challenges are a consequence of vaccine clinic models, where understandably busy, stretched healthcare personnel are trying to quickly deliver a high volume of injections to many persons with needs. Many health market settings lack flexibility in time and people sufficient for real informed assent or consent conversations about many healthcare practices. Some of this, though, reflects disinterest and defensive posturing, a lack of enculturated professional respect for patient and parent autonomy in discourse perhaps in part because of fear of the actual autonomy which they have if they choose to exercise it.

This is far from the first time that healthcare providers have created challenges in patient care by unwittingly helping to construct an environment inviting problematic approaches. My own community of Infectious Diseases sub-specialists had a long fight against the treatment of patients with antibacterial therapy for years for what has been called chronic Lyme disease. This had real consequences for patients, who naturally experienced anticipated adverse effects of long-term antibacterial therapy use and central venous access. Today we would assert the potential contribution to community-level threats of worsened bacterial drug resistance. However, that extreme approach was supported by my community's lag in recognizing that the patient experience after Lyme disease was not always wellness, and that more needed to be understood about what happens in some patients over time after they have had such an infection.

The tick-borne Lyme disease experience carries other lessons for this situation. Many people are not aware that there was encouraging medical literature on vaccine performance against Lyme disease—albeit for short-term protection. There are several likely reasons for it not showing on immunization schedules in endemic areas. Its performance characteristics made broad application to population-level recommendations challenging. If not broadly applying it, it is difficult to design and fund a supply chain for it. Yet, the surprise some people might feel from this news reflects the inherent mysticism in the process that result in the health marketplace. Even for those of us well acquainted with vaccine development and public health decision making, the nuances of this become dizzying. All of this is not conducive to an environment of transparency and broad trust, making radical conversations easier to initiate.

We are victims of our success. Instead of pushing for vaccines with astonishingly clear and compelling data, such as against measles, our thresholds for what it means to have a protected population are higher, and the system advocates strongly for protection against threats new to our consciousness and less understood by the public to be universal. While commendable, this has harms for messaging vigilance against historical threats. This is a new social mobilization frontier, one that should be met by more than a reflection on messaging, rather with critical examination of how we come to and communicate such decisions, and in what ways patients, their communities, and healthcare providers participate in both choice and adherence. Measles is Bad.

Follow the money (or, health is not all about health)

Too often, even when facing emergencies, we think about health issues as separate from needed investments in basic community infrastructure. The health business cases for what we do and why we do it often keep health separate from the rest of needs for international investment and engagement towards building more resilient communities. The thoughts here started with a collection plate.

While Liberia has its own currency, like many other economies U.S. dollars often are used. As my youngest daughter placed a bill I brought home from that trip atop a mound of domestic bills, the difference was striking. In contrast, our bill was faded, barely green and difficult to read. Part of it had been mended by a piece of tape. Small thumb sized areas were completely rubbed away. It was decorated with dirt. Having infusions of cash is not enough. Money in the U.S. is shepherded by tax, regulatory, banking and merchant interests and trust. Our cash experiences a managed life cycle that is possible only through substantial capital investments in systems that help structure how the economy works and guide the rules for participation. Aging cash is replaced. Financial systems and the ways that people interact with them are reinforced. Much of this does not exist in places in need. I have traveled many times into developing markets and had not stopped to think about this difference in the condition of paper money and what it might portend regarding the narrow nature of investments we make, and the limited investments in systems even when flushed with cash that those who live there make.

My usual work is in biomedical research and public health. We might spend many thousands of dollars delivering technology. While we try to identify local staff, train them, provide maintenance service contracts and other infrastructure, we often find it difficult to deal with deeper system issues that allow mechanisms for renewal and durable impact. We buy training but not workforce management. We buy labor hours but only in limited ways the capability to move workers to and from work sites and communicate with them such as with mobile devices and SIM cards. We also tend not to consider the myriad components of health services and their delivery that are necessary to be in place in order to make use of that equipment in meeting our mutual objectives. In short, focused health interventions fueled by cash suffer similar gaps in systems. The way that grant budgets are organized often exacerbates this. In our own funding in the U.S. for biomedical research, we often draw artificial distinctions in lanes or categories of work. Even when the intended work is narrow and not necessarily multi-disciplinary, while it is possible to charge an administrative overhead to cover some system costs, they are tokens only when working in environments that have never been capitalized initially to build those systems. This challenge is compounded when working in fragile places where strife or disease has eroded previous capital.

There are challenges, too, in both health investments and cash with regards to who wants which investments and why. For instance, when changing money in Africa, most places do not want my twenty-dollar bill. Twenty dollars matters in my household. But, if I am able to exchange it for local currency in some places, I often get a lower exchange rate and am asked several times if I have larger bills. I always get paranoid about the intended use of the dollars I relinquish in those circumstances—how they might be applied or laundered. It may simply reflect financial conditions that are less facile. Here, twenty dollars is twenty dollars no matter how it is comprised. Although, when I was very young, I got many stinky looks when paying for milkshakes with pennies. There, twenty dollars is twenty dollars presented in a particular way that drives how that twenty dollars might be accepted, valued, and used.

When bringing health-related resources into a setting, this makes me wonder what complicated considerations my host country colleagues must make on whether to accept and how to be able to use the resources; what having them might mean to their other work; how being disparately or inconveniently resourced will impact their work with others for better or ill. Does receiving my resources push them into another administrative category that means less core ministry support? Does it obligate them to try and conduct more kinds of tests indirectly related to our work that is not supported? Does it facilitate a level of training of staff high enough that now their people will be poached by better funded groups and leave gaps in health services work?

My decisions tend to be much easier. But then, it is easier for me to have and use twenty dollars, too.

When reading Fahrenheit 451 by Ray Bradbury in the 7th grade, I learned that the future is post-apocalyptic. This was reinforced by many of the book selections driven by the peculiarly consistent reading preferences of those who teach English in middle school. At 12, I looked at my parents and thought, maybe, maybe the world will end before my generation leads. Eventually, I decided that the world has a sea of cyclical angst in which all of us swim. But, like tides, the world rises and falls, constantly, on a small and large scale, whether across a continent in a war called great, or in focused calamities of communities and families. It is the present that is apocalyptic and post-apocalyptic, always.

Unsurprisingly, for some the trailing emergency of coronavirus disease (COVID-19) is an apocalypse. Many people are bracing for, subjected to, or recovering from it and its myriad impacts. What then, is the post-apocalyptic, post-COVID-19 future?

For the U.S. after World War II, the future was boom, explosive industries and opportunities. Waves of re-organization sought workforce and technology in order to supply demands of a growing middle class. It happened this way in parts of Europe and Asia, too, governments permitting, but more slowly, having more debris to remove before they could cover the same ground with fresh concrete. World War I had a different legacy. The way my elders told it, it was more local, with some communities having few return home and the towns themselves falling into memory, while others thrived, and a transient boom foretold the Great Depression. The U.S. casualties in both events were large, but those in WWII were three times greater. What recovery looks like, the post-apocalyptic stage, can be hard to predict. Ironically, I am writing this essay just after WWII's Victory in Europe (VE) day. The U.S. deaths from COVID-19 by some accounts exceed those of WWI by several fold. They are approaching ten-fold the combined U.S. total from Vietnam and Korea. Like veterans of these wars and their families, COVID-19 survivors and others impacted have durable harms.

War and pestilence, the two alike apocalyptic horsemen. Together, they remind us that not just patients and hospitals but everyone has a new world during and after such events. Early in the pandemic, I asked my adolescent children what they thought the post-COVID-19—or at least the post-initial wave—world would be like.

· Cats will be our new overlords, led by their own cat

· Places will vary in whether they keep social distancing and hand washing; some people will not understand that bacteria and viruses are still around after COVID-19

· Entering the workforce will be very difficult for them [Generation Z and younger]

· Many businesses will disappear, but with less money people will focus on the few brands they trust. Those will get larger and starting new businesses harder

In addition to recognizing that they would receive our debt and uncertainty, they struck on the idea of enculturation. What will be enculturated in recovery? Whether an event is painful enough to effect durable change or so painful that it is discounted afterwards is muddled. Seasonal influenza kills tens of thousands of people a year and the attributable mortality would be higher if we were better at counting it. We notice that disruption less. The 2009-10 H1N1 pandemic was very visible in society, and yet its lessons had minimal impact on how we initially approached SARS-CoV-2. Though, some innovations stuck. International cooperation improved after H1N1 and made it easier for coordination during the Ebola epidemic that remains active now, such as the work pushing vaccine development by CEPI. Domestic policies that evolved during H1N1 made it more likely that Ebola would trigger established regional isolation care centers and coordinated national training.

Ideally, policies enable local action. Local action happens by community members— enculturation looks different at that level. Most visibly now it is seen in masks worn on the streets, in the stores and workplaces during case count rises. This is an old habit in some parts of Asia, most notably Japan, where politeness including with respect to respiratory disease is almost a point of honor. Their COVID-19 numbers seem to have been lower than others. Though, there is some debate on that. Sometimes the lessons we learn are driven by our ability to recover. How all of that will play in areas of the world where we customarily work but did not directly support during this emergency is an open question—we largely retreated from global health roles during the pandemic. Hopefully, local innovation and mind for business and economy will have won in those locales. Vendors will create adaptive markets. And, patients would sort their own risk communication and approaches that sustain them. Our idea of critical infrastructure may evolve, acknowledging the energy and bandwidth requirements of telework. Telework may be more accepted and ebb and flow with seasons of disease. Though, we may best know the post-apocalyptic world from COVID-19 when reflecting on it and its contributions and failings during the next apocalypse.

About the Author

David Brett-Major is a U.S. internal medicine and infectious diseases physician. A retired naval officer, he served at sea and later as a medical officer in clinical, academic, and public health roles. From 2012 through 2014, he was assigned by the Navy to the WHO as a technical staff member on health security issues. In 2014, he deployed with WHO into the EVD epidemic in West Africa as a clinical consultant to Guinea, Sierra Leone, and Nigeria. He continues to work as a clinician and physician scientist, including on issues of community resilience through proactive risk management, and intersections of clinical care, public health and science necessary to manage severe emerging infections.

Related Information from the Author and Colleagues

David's indexed scientific literature can be found on PubMed, the U.S. National Library of Medicine's on-line service at http://www.ncbi.nlm.nih.gov/pubmed/?term=brett-major. Related literature can be found by selecting similar articles in individual entries.

Letter to the Adadevoh Health Trust

10 October 2015

Board of Trustees, Dr. Ameyo Stella Adadevoh Health Trust

45 Saka Tinubu Street, 2nd Floor

Victoria Island, Lagos

Nigeria

Dear Dr. Ama Adadevoh and fellow trustees,

Thank you very much for the high honor of both an invitation to your inaugural event and the receipt of the first Dr. Ameyo Stella Adadevoh Award. While I am unable to attend your October 20 event, I will be thinking of your sister and your work ahead on that day.

When I met Dr. Ameyo Adadevoh, she sat in the back of an ambulance, febrile and annoyed that she could not return home immediately and perhaps to work, distrustful of a clinical setting that was not her own and certainly not as technically appointed as she probably typically insisted. She already was several days into the course of her Ebola virus infection, moving hesitantly and suffering other severe, systemic effects. She was obviously a bright woman who interacted warmly and easily with people. Dr. Adadevoh insisted on being told the complete truth. Even though engaging in conversation let alone a technical discussion was very difficult for her at that point, I could not help feeling that in some ways I was a junior physician again, briefing a very patient teaching attending physician. Her few words were always encouraging. Dr. Adadevoh's family was attentive and caring, reflecting her nature. Soon, as news of her admission spread among the other patients, almost all of whom were her students or colleagues, her value as a friend and mentor was clear. Many of the public health response team members also had been taught by Dr. Adadevoh. They were deeply invested in her welfare. When ultimately Nigerian physicians took up care of Ebola virus disease patients, these new and older physicians alike had been her students. Some of them later went to other countries in the outbreak to be part of the regional response.

For these reasons, I think that the mission of your trust is most apt. Even from my short experience with Dr. Ameyo Adadevoh, I believe that she must have been an excellent physician. To have taught her students the lessons they carried, she believed strongly in the physician-patient relationship. She committed herself to mentoring those with her and following her. In short, she believed that health outcomes are accomplished through people. It speaks to an understanding that whatever the technology or social circumstances it is *people* who are most important. People must be present over time, connected to the mission, resourced as able, and allowed to accomplish what they believe to be right.

In future outbreaks of severe emerging infectious diseases, this will remain an essential need. Equipping all aspects of communities to serve their roles in preventing disease, caring for themselves and others, and staying together as communities is equally important. ***I have been fortunate to work for and with many people who have these aims, without whom our work in Lagos and other locations would not have been possible.***

Thank you for the Dr. Ameyo Stella Adadevoh Award. I am humbled by it and the opportunity to witness the start of your effort. Congratulations to the Trust and the community that it seeks to benefit.

Best wishes,
D.M. Brett-Major

Made in the USA
Monee, IL
08 November 2026

67379953R00163